Quick
Reference
Guide for

PAEDIATRIC
EMERGENCIES
Seizing the Golden Hours

D1494242

PAEDIAT
EMERGEN
Seizing the Gold

Claudine De Munter

editor

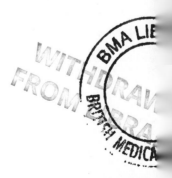

Imperial

ICP

Published by

Imperial College Press
57 Shelton Street
Covent Garden
London WC2H 9HE

Distributed by

World Scientific Publishing Co. Pte. Ltd.

5 Toh Tuck Link, Singapore 596224

USA office: 27 Warren Street, Suite 401-402, Hackensack, NJ 07601

UK office: 57 Shelton Street, Covent Garden, London WC2H 9HE

Library of Congress Cataloging-in-Publication Data
De Munter, Claudine, author.
    Quick reference guide for paediatric emergencies : seizing the golden hours / Claudine
De Munter.
        p. ; cm.
    Includes bibliographical references and index.
    ISBN 978-1-78326-450-6 (pbk. : alk. paper)
    I. Title.
    [DNLM: 1. Child. 2. Emergency Treatment--methods--Handbooks.
3. Adolescent. 4. Emergencies--Handbooks. 5. Emergency Medicine--methods--
Handbooks. 6. Infant. WS 39]
    RJ370
    618.92'0025--dc23

                                        2014021217

British Library Cataloguing-in-Publication Data
A catalogue record for this book is available from the British Library.

Printed in Singapore

CONTENTS

Contents

Contents

AUTHORS

St Mary's Hospital Imperial College Healthcare
NHS Trust, CATS (Children Acute Transport Service),
The Royal Brompton Hospital and
Imperial College London.

Specialists in the following paediatric sub-specialties:

A&E Medicine: Ian Maconochie*, Rebecca Salter
Allergy: Claudia Gore, Robert Boyle, John Warner*
Anaesthesia: Sabeena Qureshi
Cardiac Intensive Care: Margarita Burmester*
Child and Adolescent Psychiatry: Sharon Taylor
Diabetology: Samir Wassouf, Mando Watson
General Paediatrics: Nelly Ninis, Andrea Goddard, Mando Watson, Michael Coren, Michael Carter (trainee in paediatrics)
Haematology: Leena Karnik, Subarna Chakravorty
Infectious Diseases: Hermione Lyall*, Sam Walters, Shunmay Yeung, Jethro Herberg, Beate Kampmann*, Simon Kroll*, Michael Levin*, Alasdair Bamford (trainee in paediatric infectious diseases)
Intensive Care: Claudine De Munter, Mehrengise Cooper, Ruchi Sinha, Padmanabhan Ramnarayan*, David Inwald*, Simon Nadel*, Parviz Habibi*
Microbiology: Marianne Nolan
Nephrology: Jane Deal
Neurology: Leena Mewasingh

<u>Respiratory Medicine:</u> Parviz Habibi*
<u>Surgery:</u> Shamshad Syed, Munther Haddad, Sally Tenant (orthopaedics).

*Hermione Lyall, Chief of Service for Paediatrics; John Warner, Professor of Paediatrics; Beate Kampmann, Professor in Paediatric Infection & Immunity; Michael Levin, Professor in Paediatrics & International Child Health; Simon Kroll, Professor in Paediatrics & Molecular Infectious Diseases; Parviz Habibi, Reader in Paediatric Intensive Care & Respiratory Medicine; Simon Nadel, Reader in Paediatric Intensive Care; David Inwald, Senior Lecturer in Paediatric Intensive Care; Ian Maconochie, Lead Paediatric A&E Services; Margarita Burmester, Paediatric Intensive Care (Royal Brompton Hospital); Padmanabhan Ramnarayan, Paediatric Intensive Care at CATS & St Mary's PICU

<u>Allied healthcare professionals:</u>

<u>Outreach and Resuscitation Practitioner:</u> Anthony McKay
<u>Paediatric Pharmacy:</u> Penny Fletcher, Senior Lead Pharmacist

COMMENTS AND ACKNOWLEDGEMENTS

Aims and limitations of this booklet:

This booklet is only intended to be an '*aide-memoire*' for some of the most frequently encountered situations. It is a tool to be used by paediatricians and paediatric nurses. While every effort has been taken in preparing the content of this booklet, the authors, editor and publisher shall not be liable for any issues caused by the misuse of the document.

For more complete information and understanding:

— References can be found under the title of the chapters and at the end of the book (page 249).

— It is strongly advised to read textbooks and non-summarised clinical guidelines for a complete understanding of each topic.

Local guidelines:

Guidelines have been written taking into account local organisational issues within Imperial College Healthcare NHS Trust. The general information in these guidelines has been based on the review of the literature.

Acknowledgements:

We wish to thank COSMIC, Children of St Mary's Intensive Care charity for its help in the promotion of this handbook.

Contents reviewed by:

Consultants from St Mary's Hospital, Hermione Lyall, Mehrengise Cooper, Ian Maconochie, and Colin Green, Consultant in Paediatrics, East Kent Hospitals.
Pharmacist: Penny Fletcher.
Paediatric Nurses: Sonia Broadby, Anne Dowson, Deborah Lee, Sarah Wheatland, Susan Giles.
Doctors in training: Lucy Pickard, Alasdair Bamford.

ABBREVIATIONS

ABCDE: Airway, Breathing, Circulation, Disability, Exposure.

A&E: accident and emergency.

ANA: anti-nuclear antibodies.

ANCA: anti-neutrophil cytoplasmic antibody.

Anti-GBM: anti-glomerular basement membrane.

ARF: acute renal failure.

ASO(T): anti-streptolysin O (titer).

AVPU: Alert, responds to Voice, responds to Pain, Unresponsive.

BD: base deficit.

BLS: basic life support.

BM: blood glucose monitoring.

BMT: bone marrow transplant.

BNF(C): British National Formulary (for Children).

BP: blood pressure.

CATS: Children's Acute Transport Service.

CK: creatinine kinase.

CO: carbon monoxide.

CPAP: continuous positive airway pressure.

CPR: cardiopulmonary resuscitation.

CRP: C reactive protein.

CRT: capillary refill time.

Cryo: cryoprecipitates.

CSF: cerebro-spinal fluid.

CT: computed tomography.

CV: cardiovascular.

CVL: central venous line.

DC shock: direct current shock for cardioversion or defibrillation.

DIC: disseminated intra-vascular coagulation.

DKA: diabetic ketoacidosis.

DVT: deep vein thrombosis.

ECG: electrocardiography.

EMD: electrical mechanical dissociation; PEA.

ENT: ear-nose-throat.

ESR: erythrocyte sedimentation rate.

$ETCO_2$: end-tidal CO_2.

ETT: endotracheal tube.

FBC: full blood count.

FFP: fresh frozen plasma.

Fib: fibrinogen.

FiO_2: inspired fraction of oxygen.

GCS: Glasgow Coma Score.

GFR: glomerular filtration rate.

GI: gastrointestinal.

GN: glomerulonephritis.

HAS 5% or 20%: human albumin solution; 5g/100ml or 20g/100ml.

HDU: high dependency unit.

HR: heart rate.

I:E inspiratory/expiratory ratio.

iT: inspiratory time.

IUGR: intra uterine growth retardation.

IVIG: intravenous immunoglobulin.

KPa: kilo Pascal.

LP: lumbar puncture.

LMW heparin: low molecular weight heparin.

M,C&S: microscopy, culture and sensitivity.

Microgr: microgram.

MRSA: methicillin resistant *Staphylococcus aureus.*

NAI: non-accidental injury.

Nanogr: nanogram.

NG: nasogastric tube.

NICU: neonatal intensive care.

NPA: naso-pharyngeal aspirate.

NS: nephrotic syndrome.

NSAID: non-steroidal anti-inflammatory drug.

OG: orogastric tube.

PC: packed red blood cells.

PCR: polymerase chain reaction.

PCV: packed cell volume.

PEA: pulseless electrical activity = EMD.

PEEP: positive end expiratory pressure.

PICU: paediatric intensive care unit.

PIP: peak inspiratory pressure.

Plat: platelets.

PMH: past medical history.

PO_2, PCO_2: oxygen or carbon dioxide partial pressure.

PRN: pro re nata; or = as needed.

PVL: Panton–Valentine leukocidin.

Qc: cardiac output.

RICP: raised intracranial pressure.

RR: respiratory rate.

SaO_2: oxygen saturation level.

SIADH: syndrome of inappropriate ADH secretion.

SV: stroke volume.

SVT: supraventricular tachycardia.

TB: tuberculosis.

U&Es: urea, creatinine, electrolytes.

US: ultrasound.

UTI: urinary tract infection.

VF: ventricular fibrillation.

VSD: ventricular septal
    defect.
VT: ventricular
    tachycardia.

X-match: cross-match.

tds: three times a day.
bd: twice a day.
qds: four times a day.
hrly, sec, min, h, d, w, m, y:
hourly, second, minute,
    hour, day, week,
    month, year.

PO, SC, IM, IO, IV, PR:
    per oral,
    sub-cutaneous,
    intramuscular,
    intra-osseous,
    intravascular,
    per rectal.

SPOTTING THE ILL CHILD/
PATHOPHYSIOLOGY/MONITORING

LIMITING ERRORS IN THE MANAGEMENT
OF EMERGENCIES
Claudine De Munter

If a child presents with an acute problem that requires urgent management, DO NOT START WITH A DIAGNOSIS IN MIND otherwise this might mislead you and you might make the wrong therapeutic decisions.
DO A PROBLEM LIST FIRST and address EACH issue.
See further example.

DO A PROBLEM LIST IMMEDIATELY AS YOU ASSESS:

When a patient arrives acutely unwell, whilst the various organ systems are assessed through the history-taking and the initial physical examination (page 9), a PROBLEM LIST needs to be immediately created, starting with ABCD (Airway, Breathing, Circulation, Disability).

PATHOPHYSIOLOGICAL EXPLANATIONS:

For each PROBLEM on the list, think of the appropriate PATHOPHYSIOLOGICAL explanations.
This will help when deciding on the best initial management strategy.

INITIAL TREATMENT AND MANAGEMENT of the patient consists of treating the various problems identified according to the pathophysiology that explains them best.

Prioritise treatment according to ABCD: **Page 11.**

A LIST OF DIFFERENTIAL DIAGNOSIS is created in the order from the likeliest to the most unlikely during the initial management with the help of the various diagnostic tests. Targeted treatment to a diagnosis only starts now.

Example:

An 18-month-old child of African origin comes to A&E after a convulsion at home. He is coryzal, coughing, not feeding well, generally grumpy. Parents are worried. They say he has been 'hot'. On arrival, the child is uncooperative, crying. His examination seems unremarkable though he cannot be examined fully. Temperature is 38 °C. His RR is 40. HR is 140/min. The gas is normal except for Na 148 mmol/L and Hb 7 g/dL. BM is normal. The child is sent home with a diagnosis of febrile convulsion and a viral illness. He comes back a day later in status epilepticus. Though the diagnosis of febrile convulsion is the most likely, if a PROBLEM LIST had been thought through initially, the child would have undergone further tests and a decision to treat may have been made.

Start off with a problem list:

Convulsion: Short duration, seems normal afterwards. Temperature/cough/coryzal/not feeding/irritable/agitated/ raised Na on gas/anaemia on gas/tachycardia and tachypnoea/incomplete physical examination.

What are possible pathophysiological explanations?

— **Convulsion:** Febrile convulsion, meningoencephalitis, sickle cell neurological crisis, toxins, space occupying lesion, malaria, low Ca^{2+} or Na^+ levels, low BM ...

— **Cough/coryzal/temperature:** Viral/bacterial, upper or lower airway? Can't be clearly identified on examination of patient.

— **If lung disease:** Viral? Bacterial? Pneumonia? Sickle cell chest crisis? Aspiration?

— **Not feeding:** Too unwell? Social/behavioural issues? Abdomen?

— **Highish Na:** Dehydrated? Excess Na intake?

— **Anaemia:** Low iron? Sickle cell? Blood loss? Haemolysis?

— **Tachycardia, tachypnoea:** Temperature? Sepsis? Pain? Agitated?

— **Irritable/agitation:** Unwell? Pain? Social/behavioural?

— **Pain: Where?** Head? Throat? Sickle cell? Abdomen? Limbs?

— **Incomplete physical examination: further tests needed:** Chest X-ray? SaO_2? Blood tests?

— **Travel history has not been taken:** Malaria? Tuberculosis?

Conclusion: It is clear that the diagnosis of 'febrile convulsion' is not the only possible diagnosis. The child cannot be sent home on the basis that a 'febrile convulsion' is the most likely cause. Further tests and history-taking must be done to exclude other causes.

This particular child had bacterial meningitis and raised intracranial pressure by the time it was diagnosed the following day.

IN-HOSPITAL RESUSCITATION
Modified from: Resuscitation Council, 2010,
www.resus.org.uk

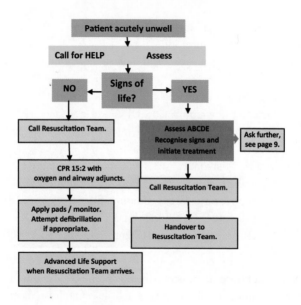

Ruling out a life-threatening condition

Ask yourself: "Is there enough evidence to know <u>for certain</u> that this is NOT a potentially life-threatening problem?"

The following is a list of common rapidly life-threatening disorders:

— Acute respiratory failure.
— Upper airways obstruction.
— Lung/lower airways obstruction. Infection. Effusion. Pneumothorax.
— Cardiac failure. Obstructive. Restrictive. Duct-dependent. Pulmonary oedema. Arrhythmia. Myocarditis.
— Septicaemia. Severe sepsis.
— Compensated shock. Decompensated shock.
— Shock with meningitis.
— Toxic shock +/− rash.
— Anaphylaxis +/− upper airway, lower airway, rash, shock.
— Raised intracranial pressure (ICP). Neurosurgical problems.
— Meningitis. Encephalitis.
— Acute metabolic decompensation.
— Severe DKA.
— Acute abdominal surgical disorder.
— Urinary/renal infection.
— Severe electrolytic derangements.

And ask yourself if what you know of the history is enough to rule out a serious life-threatening condition.

Example: **Vomiting: A tricky sign!**

History of vomiting (±minimal diarrhoea) and low grade temperature: Ask yourself if this is due to gastroenteritis. Or is the problem elsewhere? RICP? Otitis media? Upper airways? Lung? Heart dysfunction? Urine infection? Abdominal problem? Septicaemia/sepsis? Toxic shock?

Has the patient been fully examined? Is the history-taking complete?
Is more information needed? Gas? Electrolytes? BM? Blood culture? Urine sample? Other culture? U&Es, FBC, CRP? Is an LP needed? Is it safe?
X-ray? CT? US? ECG?
Do you need more help?
Is there any treatment to start that could be helpful until more is known?
Oxygen? Fluids? Antibiotics?

ASSESSING A PATIENT IN AN EMERGENCY: IMMEDIATE ACTIONS
Claudine De Munter

A airway, B breathing, C circulation, D disability, E exposure
As you approach, a quick look and listen around gives vital information on what organ systems are affected (ABCDE).
LISTEN: 1sec to gather the following immediate information:
Is the patient making noises?   ABCD?
Do you hear breathing sounds (**stridor, wheeze, grunt**)?   ABC?
Do you hear monitor sounds: SaO_2? HR?   ABC?
LOOK: 1 sec to look around:
Are there the right helpers around the patient? Is there a leader?

DO A PROBLEM LIST... NEED HELP?

Move on or take action.
Always reassess.

Any immediate actions needed?
Identify the people you will need.

As you come closer, a rapid look at the patient gives further information on organ systems ABCDE.
LOOK: **5 sec needed for first rapid clinical assessment.**
What is the patient's skin colour?   ABC?
What is the patient's activity and movements?   ABCD?
Look at respiratory movements (**chest symmetry?**).   AB?
Look at monitoring: SaO_2, HR, BP, ECG trace.   ABCD?
<u>Glance</u> at pupil. Assess AVPU scale.   CD?
<u>Glance</u> at the abdomen – is it distended?   E?

DO A PROBLEM LIST:

Any immediate actions to stabilise ABCDE?

AB	O_2, airway position, suction?
	Is the stomach empty?
	Bag and mask?
C	Obtain BP if not measured.
D	Position? Stomach empty?
ABCD	IV/IO; immediate drugs?
CD	Obtain a BM?

Move on or take action and always reassess.

Move on or take action and always reassess.

Assess ABCDE. What organ systems are affected?

TOUCH: **20 sec for rapid physical examination.**

Feel pulses (central and peripheral).	C?
Is the patient reacting?	ABCD?
What is the central/skin temperature?	ABC?
5 seconds for CRT.	ABCD?
Feel the liver.	ABC?
Feel the fontanelle.	D?
<u>Detailed</u> **look at** eyes/pupils.	D?
Examine the abdomen **if it is distended.**	E?

Move on
or
take action and
always reassess.

DO A PROBLEM LIST: Any immediate actions needed?

Move on
or
take action and
always reassess.

AB: O₂? Suction? Is the stomach empty?
    Position of patient to open airway? Bag & mask?
ABC: Position of patient to improve circulation? CPR?
C: IV/IO? Immediate drugs? Regular BP monitored?
ABCD: Gas? BM, Hb, electrolytes (Na, K, Ca), lactate, BD,
    other blood tests?
Further help?

Assess ABCDE. What organ systems are affected?

LISTEN **30 sec for further physical examination.**

Breathing sounds **(stridor, wheeze?).**	AB?
Auscultation of lung, heart.	ABC?
Listen to abdominal sounds.	E?

Move on
or
take action and
always reassess.

DO A PROBLEM LIST: Any immediate actions?

Move on
or
take action and
always reassess.

AB: O₂? Suction? Is the stomach empty?
Position of patient to open airway? Bag & mask?
ABC: Position of patient to improve circulation? CPR?
C: IV/IO? Immediate drugs? Regular BP monitored?
ABCD: Gas? BM, Hb, electrolytes (Na, K, Ca), lactate, BD,
other blood tests?
Further help?

LOOK, LISTEN, TOUCH
Complete examination.
Thoracic expansion, ribs, auscultation.
Abdominal examination, ENT, limbs.
Eyes, pupils, reflexes.

Further steps:
stabilisation,
diagnosis,
treatment.

MONITORING AND INITIAL
HELPFUL PROCEDURES
Claudine De Munter

Monitoring:

— Oxygen saturation SaO_2 and HR. If required, they need to be monitored continuously.
— BP might need to be measured every 2–5 minutes.
— ECG trace to detect arrhythmias or electrical mechanical dissociation (EMD) = pulseless electrical activity (PEA).
— Clinical reassessments needed as often as the situation requires.

Oxygen and ventilation:

— Nasal oxygen cannula cannot be used if more than 4 L/min are needed.
— If there is an oxygen mask, set the flow meter to 15 L/min.
— A simple oxygen mask delivers no more than an FiO_2 0.4.
— A mask with a reservoir bag delivers a higher FiO_2 at a flow of 15 L/min.
— The Ambu bag must be compressed when used to open the internal valve.
— Ventilation: Choose a proper-sized face mask and an Ambu bag. Make sure it is connected to oxygen and that the flow meter is at 15 L/min.
— It is rare not to be able to improve oxygenation with bag valve mask ventilation. If the chest does not rise, the patient's head must be repositioned. The bagging

technique will only be successful when the chest rises whatever the pressures required. The rate must be the physiological rate for age.

— If none of the equipment is readily available, the BLS protocol may need to be started while waiting for equipment.

— Acute RICP: If highly suspected, ventilate to low normal CO_2 (blood gas).

Position: Positioning the patient correctly is essential.

— Airway opening manoeuvres as described in BLS protocol.

— Breathing: Work of breathing can improve when sitting the patient up.

— Cardiac failure: Sitting up helps the cardiopulmonary circulation.

— Neurology: Post-ictal, the recovery position reduces risks of aspiration.

— In case of RICP: Lying the patient at 30° with head in midline position helps to assist in reducing the pressure by aiding venous drainage.

— Trauma: Positioning for cervical spine protection is fundamental.

Abdomen:

Monitoring abdominal distension is fundamental for the respiratory and haemodynamic status. Bagging will distend the stomach. Abdominal distension may also be a sign of serious GI disorder. Feeling the liver edge is useful in the presence of lung hyper-expansion, cardiac dysfunction, hypervolaemia, liver disease. A high lactate level may give information as to the presence of necrotic gut.

Last meal/NG or OG tube:

Any patient breathing with difficulty or unconscious is at risk of aspiration. Obtain information about feeding within the 4 hours prior to the emergency. Ongoing feeds need to be stopped. A naso-gastric tube (or oro-gastric in case of head trauma) will need to be placed but without causing nausea and vomiting. If ventilating with a bag and mask, the stomach distends and a gastric tube is needed for the stomach to be decompressed regularly by a helper.

Suction:

The airway of the patient may need to be suctioned to allow oxygen to be delivered more efficiently or before using bag valve mask ventilation. A blocked nose can cause serious airway obstruction in small infants. Also, think of secretions in the back of the throat. Or has the patient vomited?

IV/IO:

IV access is needed if the patient is clearly unwell. The IO access allows for <u>any drug</u> to be delivered. It is a central line but it may block rapidly and cannot be relied upon for longer than the initial phase of resuscitation and stabilisation after which reliable IV access is essential. The laboratory needs to know if blood samples are taken from the bone marrow.

Blood gas and blood tests:

Gas and glucose (BM)? pH? CO_2? Base deficit? Lactate? Hb? Often gas machines also measure levels of Na^+, K^+, Ca^{2+}. Abnormal levels of glycaemia, Na^+, K^+, Ca^{2+} can have serious negative effects on the cardiovascular and neurological systems. The result of a gas helps decide on how to adjust ventilation, fluid intake, use of inotropes, levels of glycaemia and electrolytes, needs for transfusion.

SOME TRICKY SIGNS
Claudine De Munter

Is it the wrong diagnosis?

Patients are admitted with a presumed diagnosis await-
ing confirmation. The presumptive diagnosis/level
of severity may be wrong or may change. Signs may
develop that do not correspond to the initial diagnosis/
level of severity.

Clinical parameters interpreted within the clinical
context:

Temperature, SaO_2, HR, RR, BP may seem normal according to tables but they may be abnormal within a particular
clinical context and pathophysiological process. This must
always be kept in mind when interpreting these numbers
and the way they change with time.

Pallor:

Vasoconstriction in compensated/decompensated shock?
Anaemia? Severe pain? High ICP? Vasovagal? Cold?

Low oxygen saturations (SaO_2):

A low level due to a technical problem with the probe is
frequent and must never be accepted. Correct measurements must be obtained. Levels can drop in respiratory or
cardiac dysfunction, or in shock. Feel pulses! You may need
SaO_2 in the upper right and lower limbs (page 83–88).

Rapid respiratory rate:

Know the rates as they vary with age (pages 21, 23). Sepsis? Compensated metabolic acidosis? Respiratory problem? Neurological? Pain? Heart failure? Shock?

Increased work of breathing:

Weak patients with muscle disorders who are in respiratory distress may not be able to increase the work of breathing and signs of respiratory failure can be minimal and difficult to notice. RR will usually be increased.

Upper/lower airway obstruction:

An RR may be present but there may be no air flow; check airflow from airways (feel patient's breath on your cheek, see mist in mask, listen).

Heart rate:

Variations can be due to several factors. Assess HR within the clinical context. Qc=HRxSV (Qc cardiac output, HR heart rate, SV stroke volume).

Tachycardia:

Know the rates as they vary with age (pages 21, 23). Decide if HR seems (in)appropriately high compared to the rate expected with the degree of temperature or the level of agitation or compared to the rate expected with the presumed diagnosis.

Bradycardia:

Know the rates as they vary with age (pages 21, 23). Decide if HR seems (in)appropriately low compared to the rate expected with the degree of temperature or the level of agitation or compared to the rate expected with the presumed diagnosis.

Abnormal BP:

Know the normal values as they vary with age (pages 21, 23). Never accept that the values/lack of measurement may be due to a technical problem though these can be quite frequent. <u>Measurements must be obtained</u>. <u>Feel pulses!</u> You may need BP in upper and lower limbs (page 83).

CVS:

A complete clinical assessment includes: SaO_2, <u>pulses</u>, CRT, HR, BP, liver, heart (gallop, murmur), lungs (shunts? pulmonary oedema?), CNS (hypoxaemia? RICP?), blood gas (pH, lactate, base deficit). Urine output must be measured as soon as possible. It is fundamental to interpret values within the clinical context and pathophysiological process (**pages 9–21**).

EMD (= PEA):

In EMD, there is an ECG on the monitor but no pulses to feel. This is equivalent to cardiac arrest. BP and SaO_2 are unrecordable. If SaO_2 and BP cannot be measured, this is not due to a technical error but to the loss of cardiac output. <u>Feel pulses!</u>

Prolonged capillary refill time:

Hypovolaemia? Shock? Local vascular problems? Pain? RICP? DKA? Cold ambient temperature?

Cold extremities:

Hypovolaemia? Shock? Local vascular problems? Pain? RICP? DKA? Cold ambient temperature?

AVPU/GCS score:

A good AVPU/GCS score is reassuring but does not exclude haemodynamic instability. The brain stays protected for long despite profound shock. Monitoring the neurology also includes feeling the fontanelle and looking at pupils early on and regularly during resuscitation.

TRAFFIC LIGHT SYSTEM: IDENTIFYING RISKS OF SERIOUS ILLNESS

Modified from: http://www.nice.org.uk/nicemedia/live/11010/30525/30525.pdf

This guide is valid for children under the age of 5 years old. In any situation where there is worry, a qualified clinician must assess and address the situation. The minimum that must be done by a clinician to all patients particularly when they are past 'Green boxes' includes a full examination with SaO_2, RR, HR, BP, temperature, blood gas, BM, FBC, CRP, U&Es, other blood tests, cultures and X-rays as appropriate.

Refer to the chapter 'Assessing a patient in an emergency: Immediate actions' for more detailed management in an emergency (page 9).

	Green – low risk
Colour	Normal colour of skin, lips and tongue.
Activity	Responds normally Content/smiles. Stays awake or awakens quickly. Strong normal cry/not crying.
Respiratory	Breathing normally, normal rate for age, no added sounds nor increased work of breathing.
Hydration	Normal skin and eyes. Moist mucous membrane.
Other	None of the amber or red symptoms or signs.

	Amber – intermediate risk	Red – high risk
Colour	Pallor reported by parent/carer.	Pale/mottled/ashen/blue.
Activity	Not responding normally to social cues. Wakes only with prolonged stimulation. Decreased activity. No smile.	No response. Appears ill. Does not wake. Does not stay awake. Weak. High-pitched cry. Continuous cry.
Respira-tory	Nasal flaring. Tachypnoea: age 6–12 months: RR > 50 breaths/minute; age > 12 months: RR > 40 breaths/minutes. SaO$_2$ ≤ 95% in air. Crackles.	Grunting. Tachypnoea: RR > 60 breaths/minute. Moderate to severe chest indrawing.
Hydration	Dry mucous membranes. Poor feeding in infants. CRT ≥ 3 seconds. Reduced urine output.	Reduced skin turgor.
Other	Fever for ≥ 5 days. Swelling of a limb or joint. Non-weight bearing limb. Not using an extremity. A new lump > 2 cm.	Age 0–3 months: temperature ≥ 38°C. Age 3–6 months: temperature ≥ 39°C. Non-blanching rash. Bulging fontanelle. Neck stiffness. Seizure. Focal neurological signs. Bile-stained vomiting.

NORMAL HEART RATE, RESPIRATORY RATE, BLOOD PRESSURE
APLS 2012: Pages 9–21 of this book

Age	Heart rate	Respiratory rate	Blood pressure
Newborn	90–180	40–60	60–90
1m	110–180	30–50	70–104
3m	110–180	30–45	70–104
6m	110–180	25–35	72–110
1y	80–160	20–30	72–110
2y	80–140	20–28	74–110
4y	80–120	20–26	78–112
6y	75–115	18–24	82–115
8y	70–110	18–22	86–118
10y	70–110	16–20	90–121
12y	60–110	16–20	90–126
14y	60–100	16–20	92–130

HEART RATE AND TEMPERATURE IN A CHILD LESS THAN 1 YEAR OLD

Modified from: Hanna, CM, Greenes, DS.
Annals of Emergency Medicine,
2004, 43(6): 699–705.

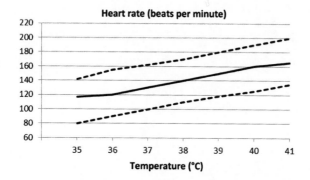

TRICKY SITUATION: A heart rate is considered abnormal when its rise is disproportionate to the rise of the temperature. Knowing how the HR rises physiologically with the temperature helps in assessing a tachycardia (page 16).

LIFE SUPPORT ALGORITHMS

PAEDIATRIC BASIC LIFE SUPPORT (BLS)
Modified from: Resuscitation Council, 2010,
www.resus.org.uk

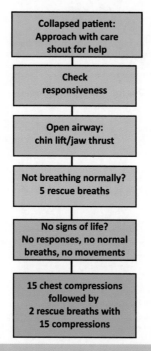

Collapsed patient:
Approach with care
shout for help

Check
responsiveness

Open airway:
chin lift/jaw thrust

Not breathing normally?
5 rescue breaths

No signs of life?
No responses, no normal
breaths, no movements

15 chest compressions
followed by
2 rescue breaths with
15 compressions

Reassess after each cycle

PAEDIATRIC ADVANCED LIFE SUPPORT (ALS)

Modified from: Resuscitation Council, 2010,

www.resus.org.uk

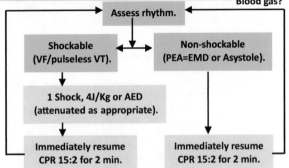

Unresponsive?

CPR 5 initial breaths then 15:2. Attach difibrillator/ monitor. Minimise interruptions to CPR.

Call Resuscitation Team after 1 min CPR if alone.

Measure BM? Blood gas?

Assess rhythm.

Shockable (VF/pulseless VT).

Non-shockable (PEA=EMD or Asystole).

1 Shock, 4J/Kg or AED (attenuated as appropriate).

Immediately resume CPR 15:2 for 2 min.

Immediately resume CPR 15:2 for 2 min.

During CPR:
-ABCD approach.
-Controlled oxygenation and ventilation.
-Attempt or verify IV/IO access.
-Give uninterrupted compressions once trachea is intubated.
-Give adrenaline 1:10000 every 3–5 min (page 217).
-Investigations.
-Correct reversible causes*.
-Treat precipitating causes.
-Temperature control.
-Therapeutic hypothermia?

*Reversible causes: hypoxia, hypovolaemia, hypokalaemia, hyperkalaemia, metabolic, hypothermia, tension pneumothorax, tamponade, cardiac, toxins, thromboembolism.

PERSONAL NOTES

RESPIRATORY

THE CHOKING CHILD
Modified from: Resuscitation Council, 2010, www.resus.org.uk

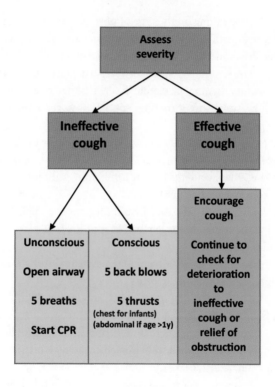

UPPER AIRWAYS OBSTRUCTION
Updated by Parviz Habibi, 2012

HELP: Depending on the type of obstruction and the clinical assessment, calling for help from anaesthetists, paediatric intensivists and ENT specialists may be necessary <u>early on</u>.

Croup: Age 3m–3y; slow onset, particularly in winter, inspiratory stridor, moderate fever, barking cough, good swallow, some sore throat, no special posture, often coryzal (page 34).

Bacterial tracheitis: Onset <24h, stridor varies (none/inspiratory/expiratory), high fever, marked coughing, septic looking. Management: Urgent intubation, antibiotics (ceftriaxone, pages 220, 226).

Retropharyngeal abscess: Inspiratory stridor, high fever, toxic, dysphonia. Management: Urgent ENT surgery, antibiotics (page 225).

Inhalation hot gases/burns: Management: Intubate early before airway swelling appears (rapidly!).

Epiglotittis: Age 1–7y, onset <24h, any season, high fever, septic/toxic looking, rasping sounds, cannot swallow, severe sore throat. Posture: Sits forwards, open mouth, drooling. Management: Urgent intubation in theatres + ceftriaxone (pages 33, 220, 226).

Foreign body: 80% of cases are under 3y, sudden onset, any season, varying stridor, no fever, some choking, some coughing, some dysphonia, swallow varies.
Management: Rigid bronchoscopy.

EPIGLOTTITIS
Updated by Parviz Habibi, 2012

Symptoms: Age 1–7y, onset <24h, <u>high fever</u>, upper airways obstruction, septic/toxic looking, drooling, sitting forwards with open mouth, rasping, cannot swallow, sore throat.

Cause: *Haemophilus influenzae* in unimmunised children, *Pneumococcus, Staphylococcus, Group A Streptococcus.*

DO: <u>Minimal handling and</u>

— Call senior help: anaesthetist and ENT and PICU teams.
— Humidified oxygen.
— Child to theatres for intubation by anaesthetist and ENT.

DO NOT:

— Do not change child's position or do oropharyngeal examination.
— Do not do IV cannula or take bloods.
— Do not upset the child or leave the child unsupervised.
— X-ray is not necessary.

Antibiotics (ceftriaxone) and other treatment: after intubation.

Once intubated: Pages 183–187.
— Antibiotics: broad spectrum (ceftriaxone). (Pages 220, 226.)
— Fluid bolus if haemodynamic status requires it. (Pages 47, 216.)

Transfer to a PICU.

MANAGEMENT OF CROUP
Updated by Parviz Habibi, 2012

**Leave child in a comfortable position. No tongue depressor.
No IV line or blood taking. No X-ray. Pages 9–21.**

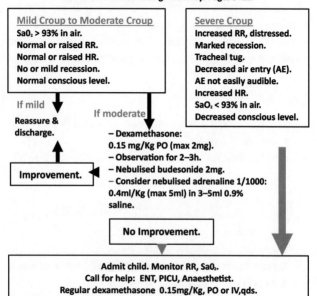

Mild Croup to Moderate Croup
SaO_2 > 93% in air.
Normal or raised RR.
Normal or raised HR.
No or mild recession.
Normal conscious level.

Severe Croup
Increased RR, distressed.
Marked recession.
Tracheal tug.
Decreased air entry (AE).
AE not easily audible.
Increased HR.
SaO_2 < 93% in air.
Decreased conscious level.

If mild
Reassure & discharge.

If moderate
– Dexamethasone:
0.15 mg/Kg PO (max 2mg).
– Observation for 2–3h.
– Nebulised budesonide 2mg.
– Consider nebulised adrenaline 1/1000:
0.4ml/Kg (max 5ml) in 3–5ml 0.9% saline.

Improvement.

No Improvement.

Admit child. Monitor RR, SaO_2.
Call for help: ENT, PICU, Anaesthetist.
Regular dexamethasone 0.15mg/Kg, PO or IV,qds.

If evidence of respiratory failure before help arrives:
1) Stay with child.
2) Nebulised adrenaline 0.4ml/Kg; 1:1000, in 3–5ml 0.9% saline.
Up to maximum of 5ml adrenaline, repeat if needed.
3) Heliox with oxygen mask or nebuliser (page 37).
4) Is bag-mask ventilation required at this stage?
5) Intubation and PICU: Intubation should be in theatres with anaesthetists and ENT surgeons.

BRONCHIOLITIS — ACUTE CARE IN HOSPITAL (BACH PROTOCOL)

Imperial NIHR Biomedical Research Centre, 2010.
Updated by Parviz Habibi, 2012

<u>Cause:</u> RSV, rhinovirus, metapneumovirus, adenovirus, parainfluenzae, enterovirus. Pertussis and mycoplasma can be associated.

<u>Do:</u> FBC, U&Es, CRP, blood gas, NPA, chest X-ray.

<u>Severe bronchiolitis:</u> Pages 9–21.

SaO_2 in air <93%, difficulty feeding, increased work of breathing. Tachypnoea >60 breaths/min. Blood gas: $PaCO_2$ normal.

Step 1:

O_2 therapy via a 3-valve face mask with reservoir bag:

— Sit up. Apply suction in nose and mouth.
— Oxygen flow rate 10L/min.
— Use warm humidification (MR850 Fisher & Paykel).
— Use a bonnet/hat to keep face mask straps on head.

Step 2:

Nebulise 4 ml of 3% saline +1.25 mg salbutamol.
— To obtain 3% saline: Use ready-made Muco Clear 3% saline nebules or prepare 1 ml NaCl 30% + 9 ml water for injection = 10 ml 3% saline.
— Nebulise at flow rate 8–10L/min.

— Give 8 hrly.
— Ensure optimal delivery: Support baby leaning forward, choose a well-sized, tight-fitting face mask held to face (+ chin lift if necessary).

Feeding/hydration support: Ensure adequate hydration. Avoid NG tubes if possible. Give small amounts and frequent bottle/breast feeds. Give IV fluids if severe respiratory distress.

Face-mask intolerant patients: Engage/encourage parents as much as possible. Use swaddling to comfort. Use a bonnet/hat to keep face mask straps on the child's head.

Assessment after 15 min

Step 3: Not clinically improved by 15 minutes:
Start Heliox + O$_2$ therapy **(see set up below):**

— Use warm humidification (MR850 Fisher & Paykel).
— Use a 3-valve face mask with reservoir bag.
— Use swaddling to comfort babies and ensure mask tolerance.
— Use a bonnet/hat to keep face mask straps on.
— Continue nebuliser therapy as above.

For greatest Heliox effect:

— Oxygen flow rate + Heliox flow rate should be equal to 10L/min.
— Use the lowest O_2 flow rate to keep SaO_2 ≥93%.
— Alter O_2 flow rates in steps of 0.5L/min.

Step up **Step down**

Heliox Flow rate L/min	Oxygen Flow rate L/min	Estimated FiO$_2$
10	0	21%
9	1	28%
8	2	35%
7	3	42%
6	4	50%
If need more than 4L/min O$_2$ to maintain Sats > 93% consider CPAP/CNEP		

Nasal cannula therapy: Use only humidified O_2 therapy via nasal cannula. Heliox therapy is not effective by nasal cannula at low flow rates.

Co-infections: If you suspect influenza, start oseltamivir.

If there are signs of bacterial superadded infection, add antibiotics as directed (pages 227, 228).

Indications for respiratory support (CPAP or intubation):

Developing signs of severity despite treatment: apnoea, dropping conscious level, exhaustion with rising $PaCO_2$ or dropping SaO_2.

— Try adrenaline nebuliser if work of breathing is efficient enough. 1:1000, 0.4 ml/Kg (max 5ml) in 3–5 ml 0.9% saline.
— Try CPAP nasal flow driver at 7 cm H_2O if this seems reasonable clinically.
— NG tube free drainage. Stop all feeds.
— Call PICU/anaesthetists.

ACUTE ASTHMA GUIDELINE:
SEVERE AND LIFE THREATENING
Updated by Parviz Habibi, 2014

Assess severity of exacerbation and always treat according to most severe features.

History: **Frequency? Routine medication? Steroids? Allergy?**

<u>SEVERE:</u> **Pages 9–21.**
Saturation <92% in air.
Too breathless to talk/eat.
RR >40/min if 2–5y, >30/min if >5y.
HR >140/min if 2–5y, >125/min if >5y.
Using accessory muscles.
Peak flow 33–50%.

Call senior help.

— High flow (≥10L/min) oxygen face mask with reservoir bag.
— Monitor SaO_2, RR, ECG, BP.
— Keep saturation >95%.
— Salbutamol via O_2 driven nebuliser: 2.5 mg preschool age, 5 mg for older patients; 3× back-to-back in first hour.
— Add Ipratropium to 2nd/3rd nebuliser: If >5y: 500 microgr; if 1–5y: 250 microgr; if <1y: 125 microgr.
— Prednisolone 2 mg/Kg, PO, or Hydrocortisone 4 mg/Kg, IV, 8 hrly.
— Continuous monitoring and assessment.

Not responding? Then treat as 'LIFE THREATENING'
(see later) while considering other diagnosis:
Pneumothorax? Collapsed lobe? Dehydration? Inadequate drug delivery? Wrong diagnosis? Anaphylaxis (page 50)?
Foreign body? Aspiration? Upper airways obstruction (page 32)? Atypical pneumonia? Cystic fibrosis?

<u>LIFE THREATENING:</u> **Pages 9–21.**
Saturation <92% in oxygen. Cyanosis.
Poor respiratory effort. Silent chest.
Agitation/Exhaustion/Reduced level of consciousness.
Hypotension.
Peak flow <33% predicted.

Activate paediatric crash call and paediatric/PICU consultant.

— High flow (≥10L/min) oxygen face mask with reservoir bag.
— Monitor SaO_2, RR, ECG, BP.
— Back-to-back nebulised salbutamol and ipratropium with 2nd and 3rd nebulisers, then 4–6 hrly.
— Hydrocortisone 4 mg/Kg IV.
— IV Salbutamol (page 215). <u>Bolus:</u> <2y: 5 microgr/Kg over 5–10 min; >2y: 15microgr/Kg (max 250 microgr) over 5–10 min. Side effects: Lactic or metabolic acidosis, tachycardia, arrhythmias, tremor, hypokalaemia, hyperglycaemia, hypophosphataemia. <u>Infusion:</u> 10 mg (= 10 ml) added to 40 ml 0.9% saline/5% dextrose, 1–5 microgr/Kg/min = 0.3–1.5 ml/Kg/h.
— Optimise hydration. Regular blood gases. Blood tests including U&Es. Give K^+ supplements for hypokalaemia if necessary (page 107).
— Chest X-ray.

30 minutes after starting the infusion:

If not responding:

— Consider double rate of salbutamol infusion.
— Aminophylline (page 216): Loading dose 5 mg/Kg (max 500 mg) over 20 min, with ECG, BP monitoring. Do not give if already taking oral theophylline. Main side effects: Arrhythmias and hypokalaemia.
— Magnesium sulphate 10% or 50% (page 216): 40 mg/Kg over 20 min, max 2g. If using a 50% solution, dilute 5 × in 0.9% saline. Beware of dropping BP!

Urgent anaesthetic opinion. Admit to PICU/HDU.

If improving:
— Continue IV bronchodilators /1 hrly nebulised salbutamol /6 hrly nebulised ipratropium /6 hrly hydrocortisone.

SICKLE CELL ACUTE CHEST SYNDROME (ACS)
Updated by Subarna Chakravorty, 2012

Symptoms:

May present as abdominal pain or develop during a painful vaso-occlusive limb crisis.

— Pain (often pleuritic): Chest wall, upper abdomen, thoracic spine.
— Dyspnoea.
— Cough may be late.
— High fever, tachypnoea, tachycardia.
— Lung consolidation: Usually bilateral, at the bases, may be unilateral. Bronchial breathing may be striking. Physical signs precede X-ray changes.

Differential diagnosis:

Sickle lung and pneumonia usually indistinguishable. Pleuritic pain may also be due to spinal/rib/sternal infarction or from sub-diaphragmatic inflammation.

Investigations:

Monitor respiratory status and SaO_2 (pages 9–21). If SaO_2 <90% in air: Do arterial blood gases, chest X-ray, cultures (blood, throat and sputum). Serology (Mycoplasma, Legionella, viral).

Group & Save; phenotype red cells for transfusion. If the diagnosis of ACS is clear: X-match blood for exchange transfusion.

Management:

Call haematology consultant and PICU.

— Oxygenation: Face mask oxygen with a reservoir bag, 15L/min.
— Low threshold for CPAP: If SaO_2 <93% in air.
— Exchange transfusion: If worsening chest X-ray, rapid fall in SaO_2 or persistent fever.
— Ventilation: Rarely required and usually due to inadequate management or late presentation.
— Intravenous fluids with hyperhydration (see references on the management of painful sickle cell crisis, local guidelines).
— Antibiotics: IV cefuroxime tds and oral clarithromycin bd.
— Incentive spirometry +/− device with physiotherapy.
— Bronchodilators: If known airways disease.
— Diuretics: Contraindicated even if X-ray mimics pulmonary oedema.

SICKLE CELL ACUTE ABDOMINAL CRISIS
Updated by Subarna Chakravorty, 2012

Symptoms:

— Insidious non-specific pain.
— Anorexia and distension.
— Reduced bowel sounds.
— Some generalised non-specific abdominal tenderness.
— Vomiting and diarrhoea: Not prominent features.

Particular case of the Girdle (or mesenteric) syndrome:
— Ileus with vomiting, silent distended abdomen, distended bowel loops and fluid levels on abdominal X-ray. Large liver.
— Often bilateral basal lung consolidation.

Investigations:

— Oxygen saturation.
— Arterial blood gas (pH, lactate), electrolytes, glucose.
— Abdominal ultrasound and X-ray. Chest X-ray.
— FBC, CRP, U&Es, liver enzymes, amylase to exclude pancreatitis.

Treatment:

— Analgesia and fluids.
— If vomiting, abdominal distension or absent bowel sounds: Give nothing by mouth and consider NG on free drainage.

— Monitor abdominal girth 1–4 hrly; measure liver size bd.
— If SaO$_2$<90% in air, see Acute Chest Syndrome protocol (above).
— Antibiotics: Pyrexial/unwell: Cefuroxime tds + Metronidazole tds.
— Girdle syndrome is an indication for exchange transfusion.

Other sickle cell crises to think of:
See references and local guidelines.

HAEMODYNAMIC/SEVERE SEPSIS/ INFLAMMATORY

HAEMODYNAMIC INSTABILITY
Claudine De Munter, Simon Nadel, 2012,
based on APLS 2012

Causes:

Severe dehydration? Haemorrhagic? Septic? Cardiac? Myocarditis (page 89)? Anaphylactic (page 50)? Toxic shock (page 57)?

Signs – Constantly reassess ABCDE: Pages 9–21.

— Pale, mottled, cold extremities, ± rash.
— AB: High RR ± chest signs. SaO_2 normal to low depending on cause and cardiac output.
— C: Disproportionately high HR. Prolonged CRT. Normal to low BP. Weak to absent peripheral pulses. Heart sounds: Normal or gallop. Liver: If increased, think of primary cardiac failure. Reduced urine output.
— D: GCS, AVPU can stay normal even if BP is very low. GCS, AVPU can also become abnormal (irritability to lethargy to unconscious) due to low BP or coexisting neurological disorder (infection? bleed?). Pupils and fontanelle must be examined initially and regularly.
— E: Any visible abnormality? Skin? Abdomen? Bone? Urinary?
— Gas: Metabolic acidosis; increased BD; normal to high lactate.
— BM low or high depending on stress response.
— ECG and troponin I to help assess myocardial function. Cardiomyopathy? Myocarditis?

<u>Treatment in the first 2 hours:</u>

— Oxygen high flow, 15 L/min, face mask with reservoir bag.
— Constantly reassess: All signs change quickly as disease or resuscitation progress. Monitor SaO_2, HR, ECG continuously and BP as often as needed.
— Control airway and call anaesthetist/PICU early (risks of pulmonary oedema).
— Fluids: See later.
— Electrolytes and BM: Correct low K^+, Ca^{2+}, low BM (pages 107, 110, 158).
— Secure vascular access: IO or IV central line.
— Intubate after 40 ml/Kg over the first 1–2 h, if the patient is still in shock (pages 183, 187).
— Inotropes: Peripheral dopamine or central IV adrenaline (page 217).
— Antibiotics: Ceftriaxone (>1 m) or cefotaxime (≤1 m) + amoxicillin (≤2 m). For other antibiotics see pages 220 and 231.
— Steroids: Debated as to the role in persistent shock.
— If anaphylaxis: **Adrenaline IM (page 50).**
— If haemorrhage: **Page 173.**
— If cardiac: **Pages 79–89. Do an ECG. Optimise electrolytes to high normal levels. Measure troponin I and CK. Call cardiologist: Echo, specific drugs, ECMO?**
— If any abnormal neurological signs appear during resuscitation: **Drop in GCS, dilated pupils, bulging fontanelle: think of RICP (page 130).**

CRYSTALLOID/COLLOID
20ml/Kg (or 10 + 10)
Assess response ↓5 min.

CRYSTALLOID/COLLOID
20ml/Kg (or 10 + 10)
Assess response ↓5 min.

CRYSTALLOID/COLLOID
20ml/Kg (or 10 +10)
Assess response ↓5 min.

— Call PICU if ≥40ml/Kg.

— Intubation if ≥40ml/Kg + ongoing shock. Beware of the side effects of induction drugs **(page 185).**

— Clotting: **Consider packed red blood cell, FFP, cryoprecipitate.**

— Antibiotics: **Page 231.**

APLS 2012 /ATLS 2008

— Coexistence of RICP? If ongoing shock after >40ml/Kg, assess clinically. If there is a possible RICP, early use of inotropes might help to maintain BP above normal with less fluids (pages 130, 218).

— Associated primary cardiac disorder? (E.g. myocarditis, page 89). Feel liver. Murmur? Arrhythmia? Start inotropes.

— Electrolyte abnormalities (low K^+, Ca^{2+}, Mg^{2+}, glucose) need correcting to optimise BP and myocardial function (pages 107, 158, 219).

— Severe DKA: Be guided by BP and the persistence of polyuria. Very careful fluid resuscitation: One fluid bolus only if shock present (BP low, no polyuria). Start insulin (pages 147, 219).

ANAPHYLAXIS

Muraro *et al.* EAACI Allergy 2007
and Resuscitation Council.
Reviewed by Claudia Gore, Robert Boyle,
John Warner, 2014

Diagnosis:

— Acute onset.
— Life-threatening ABC problems: Swelling, hoarse, stridor, drooling, wheeze, fatigue, cyanosis, confusion, agitation, pale, clammy, drowsy/coma (pages 9–21, 47).
— Profuse vomiting ± diarrhoea and abdominal pain.
— Skin rash or swellings: 80–90% of cases. But there may be no skin/mucosal changes.

Diagnosis is <u>very</u> likely if the following 3 criteria are met:

— Sudden onset and rapid progression of symptoms.
— Life-threatening ABC problems (see above).
— Skin and/or mucosal changes (flushing, urticaria, angioedema).

The following supports the diagnosis:

— Exposure to a known allergen for the patient.

Remember:

— Skin/mucosal changes alone are not a sign of anaphylactic reaction.
— Skin/mucosal changes can be subtle or absent in 20% of reactions.

— There can also be gastrointestinal symptoms (ex: vomiting, abdominal pain, incontinence).
— Shock with low BP can be the only symptom.

Management:

— Secure airway: Monitoring SaO_2, RR, HR, BP, CRT, pulses, blood gases. Signs of obstruction? Call anaesthetists, ENT, PICU early (page 32). Guedel airway? Bag-mask ventilation? Intubation?
— Remove allergen as soon as possible. Use latex-free equipment.
— Lie patient flat and raise the legs.
— IM adrenaline 1:1000: Do not delay. See page 52.
— Review A, B: High flow oxygen 15 L/min face mask with reservoir.
— Monitor SaO_2, RR, BP, HR, CRT, pulses, blood gas (pages 9–21).
— If wheeze: Inhaled/nebulised Salbutamol; repeated after 5 min. Adrenaline IM if in distress.
— If stridor: Nebulised adrenaline. Adrenaline IM if in distress. Can be repeated after 5 min.
— Angioedema/urticaria: Cetirizine PO or chlorphenamine IM/PO. Reassess.
— Hypotension/collapse: Adrenaline IM, colloid or 0.9% saline 20ml/Kg, IV/IO, hydrocortisone IV/IO, chlorphenamine IV/IO/IM. Adrenaline can be repeated after 5 min.

Further management:

— Fluid challenge: 20 ml/Kg, 0.9% saline IV/IO. Max 40 ml/Kg. Inotropes indicated ± ventilation. <u>No colloids:</u> They may cause allergic reactions.
— Cetirizine PO: If able to tolerate oral medication; see further
— Chlorphenamine IV: If not able to tolerate oral medication.
— Hydrocortisone IV: 4 mg/Kg.

If no response, continue with: — IM adrenaline every 5 min. — 0.9% saline boluses 10–20 ml/Kg if shock. — Call PICU/anaesthetists.	Obese children: Epipen needles might be too short to reach the muscle. Use a normal needle/ syringe.

No response to 3 doses adrenaline IM:
— Give adrenaline IV/IO 1:10000: 1 microgr/Kg.
— Consider infusion: 0.3 mg/Kg in 50 ml syringe 0.9% saline (page 217). Start at 0.05 microgr/Kg/min. Continuous monitoring SaO_2, RR, BP, HR, CRT, pulses, frequent blood gases.

<u>Adrenaline IM:</u> **Page 217.**

<7 Kg: Adrenaline 1:1000,0.01 ml/kg.
7–25 Kg: Epipen Junior (0.15 mg).
>25 Kg: Epipen (0.3 mg).
OR
Adrenaline IM,
  1:1000 (1 mg = 1 ml)
}
    <2y: 0.062 ml.
    2–5: 0.125 ml.
    6–11: 0.25 ml.
    >11: 0.5 ml.

Salbutamol nebulised: 5 mg (2.5 mg if <2 y) (page 215).

Salbutamol inhaled: 10 puffs via spacer.

Adrenaline nebulised: (1:1000) 0.4 ml/Kg, max 5 ml, in at least 3 ml 0.9% saline.

Cetirizine oral (oral = safe): <2 y: 0.5 mg/Kg. 2–6 y: 5 mg. >6 y: 10 mg.

Prednisolone oral (oral = safe): 2 mg/Kg (max 40 mg).

Chlorphenamine: see below

Hydrocortisone: see below

	Chlorphenamine IM, IV slow	Hydrocortisone IM, IV slow
<6 m:	250 microgr/Kg	25 mg
6 m–6 y:	2.5 mg	50 mg
6–12 y:	5 mg	100 mg
>12 y:	10 mg	200 mg

— If no cardiorespiratory signs: Observe for at least 2 h.
— If respiratory signs: Observe for at least 4 h.
— Hypotension/collapse: Admit to PICU.
— If going home, warn parents of late phase symptoms at 4–8 h.

KAWASAKI DISEASE (KD)

Management of Kawasaki disease. *Arch Dis Child*, 2014 Jan; 99(1): 74–83.

Efficacy of immunoglobulin plus prednisolone for prevention of coronary artery abnormalities in severe Kawasaki disease (RAISE study): a randomised, open-label, blinded-endpoints trial.
The Lancet, 2012, 28; 379(9826): 1613–1620.

Reviewed by Sam Walters and Michael Levin, 2014

Diagnosis:

KD must be considered in any child with a febrile illness if pyrexia persists longer than 4 to 5 days. KD affects mostly children aged 3 m to 6 y.

Diagnostic criteria: Fever >3 to 5 days PLUS 4 of 5 of the following:

1. Conjunctivitis: Bulbar, non-suppurative.
2. Lymphadenopathy: Cervical, >1.5 cm in size.
3. Rash: Polymorphous, no vesicles.
4. Lips or oral mucosa: Red cracked lips, strawberry tongue, erythema of pharynx.
5. Extremities: Erythema and oedema of palms and soles.
— These criteria may present sequentially.
— Irritability is usually present.
— Incomplete KD is possible with fewer than 4 criteria, especially in babies.

Often present:

— Erythema + induration at sites of BCG immunisation.
— Other: Arthritis, aseptic meningitis, pneumonitis, uveitis, gastroenteritis, meatitis, dysuria, otitis, gall bladder hydrops, myocarditis.
— Inflammatory markers: CRP, ESR, neutrophils are usually high. In that case, fewer than 4 criteria may be used to make a diagnosis.
— Falling Hb and albumin levels are common in severe cases.

Cardiac complications:

— Life-threatening coronary arterial aneurysms and myocarditis.
— If coronary artery *dilatations* are detected, fewer than 4 criteria may be used to establish the diagnosis.

Blood tests:

Raised acute phase proteins, neutrophilia, high CRP, high ESR, thrombocytosis (2nd week), deranged liver function, low albumin, low Hb, sterile pyuria, CSF pleocytosis (lymphocytes).

Treatment:

— Aspirin 30 mg/kg/day and IVIG 2 g/kg over 10 hours.
— Seek expert advice after one dose of IVIG if no clinical improvement and fever persists or if there are poor prognostic markers (young age, high inflammatory markers, low albumin, low Hb).

— In these severe cases: After seeking expert advice, repeat IVIG, add methyl prednisolone IV 0.8 mg/Kg/day for 5 days then oral prednisolone 2 mg/kg tailoring over 4 weeks. Consider infliximab or anakinra if no response to IVIG.

— If there are giant coronary aneurysms (above 8 mm), add heparin and warfarin (with expert advice).

— Do a heart echo initially, 2 weeks later and after 6 weeks if initially normal. Cardiologists need to be invloved early.

Convalescent phase:

— Peeling of skin fingers, soles, often thrombocytosis.

TOXIC SHOCK SYNDROME (TSS)

Principles & Practice of Pediatric Infectious Diseases,
3ʳᵈ ed., Elsevier, 2008.
Ferguson, AJ. *Lancet Infect Dis,* **2009, 9(5): 281–290.**
Reviewed by Sam Walters, 2012

Caused by a toxin producing bacteria:

If Staphylococcus: TSS can occur with a skin wound (even minor), burns, foreign bodies (vaginal tampons, nose packs).

If Streptococcus: TSS is usually linked with an invasive infection (e.g. empyema, septic arthritis, necrotising fasciitis).

Symptoms:

The diagnosis is based on the presence of:

— Shock (pages 9–21, 47).
— High fever >38.9 °C (more common with Staphylococcus).
— Flu-like illness (more common with Streptococcus).
— Diarrhoea and vomiting (more common with Staphylococcus).
— Multisystem involvement.

Plus at least 3 of the following:

— Rash: Diffuse macular erythroderma.
— Mucous membrane: Conjunctivitis (non-suppurative), red lips, 'strawberry tongue', pharyngeal erythema.
— Renal involvement.
— Haematological involvement (thrombocytopaenia).

— Hepatic involvement.
— Muscle pain (high creatinine kinase; more with Staphylococcus).
— Soft tissue: Necrotising fasciitis or myositis (more with Streptococcus).
— Encephalopathy (more common with Staphylococcus).

A history of skin wound, foreign body etc. . . facilitates the diagnosis.

Convalescence: Skin peeling after 1–2 w on palms of hand and soles of feet.

Laboratory tests:

Coagulopathy with thrombocytopenia, left shift neutrophils, multiorgan dysfunction including liver and renal, raised creatinine kinase. Identified TSST-1 producing Staphylococcus growing from mucosa or infected site or toxin producing Streptococcus from throat or from a normally sterile site.

Treatment:

— Treatment of the local wound, eliminating the source of production of toxins.
— Ceftriaxone + clindamycin (+ vancomycin if MRSA is possible). Clindamycin inhibits toxin release (page 231).
— Multiorgan support (PICU bed?) (page 47).
— IVIG 2 g/Kg over 10 hours.

MENINGOCOCCAL SEPSIS

Pollard, AJ. *Arch Dis Child*, 1999, 80: 290–296.
Pathan, N, Faust, S, Levin, M. *Arch Dis Child*, 2003,
88(7): 601–607.
http://www.hpa.org.uk/Topics/InfectiousDiseases/
InfectionsAZ
Updated by Simon Nadel and Simon Kroll, 2013

Signs:

May present with septicaemia, meningitis, or both.

— Rash: Petechial / purpuric / atypical / initially blanching (30% of cases) / absent in some cases.
— History: Short (1–2 days) starting with non-specific signs (pyrexial, vomiting, irritable, fatigue, pain in a limb).

Presenting with signs of shock: Pages 9–21, 47.

Tachypnoea, hypoxia, tachycardia, cool peripheries, long CRT, metabolic acidosis (BD>–5, lactate >2mmol/L), confusion/drowsiness, poor urine output and low BP (late sign). Call anaesthetist and PICU early.

Treatment and monitoring:

— ABC, high flow O_2 (15 L/min) face mask with reservoir bag.
— BM, blood gas, 2 IV cannulae (or IO). No LP!
— Monitor continuously: Conscious level, SaO_2, RR, HR, BP, CRT, base deficit, urine output.

— Blood tests: Glucose, FBC, CRP, Na^+, Ca^{2+}, Mg^{2+}, K^+, PO_4, lactate, urea, creatinine, clotting, X-match, blood culture, EDTA for PCR.
— NO lumbar puncture.
— Fluid: 20 ml/Kg 0.9% saline over 5–10 min. To be repeated if necessary with 0.9% saline or 4.5% human albumin solution.
— Antibiotics: Ceftriaxone (80 mg/Kg) or cefotaxime (50 mg/Kg) (page 231).

Persistent signs of shock after 40–60 ml/Kg fluid:

— Call anaesthetists: Elective intubation and ventilation (pages 47, 183, 187) if over 40 ml/Kg of fluid bolus are needed.
— Nasogastric tube. Urine catheter. Chest X-ray.
— Continue with fluid boluses over 5–10 min, as often as required.
— Inotropes: With an IV peripheral catheter, start dopamine. As soon as a CVC is obtained or an IO needle is placed, start adrenaline or noradrenaline (pages 47, 217).

Early complications that need urgent corrections:

— Pulmonary oedema (can be present at onset): early elective intubation with cuffed ETT and use PEEP (5–10 cm H_2O) (page 189).
— Hypoglycaemia, hypokalaemia, hypomagnesaemia, hypocalcaemia, acidosis: Normalising the levels stabilises BP and improves cardiac output (pages 107, 109, 110, 158, 219).
— Anaemia, coagulopathy: Give FFP, red blood cells, platelets as required.
— RICP: Page 130.

<u>Presenting with or developing RICP:</u> **Page 130.**

— ABC, high flow O_2 (15 L/min) face mask with reservoir bag.
— BM, blood gas, 2 IV cannulae (or IO). Anaesthetists/ PICU early!
— No lumbar puncture!
— Monitor continuously or regularly: Conscious level, SaO_2, RR, HR, BP, CRT, base deficit, urine output, NG tube.
— Blood tests: Glucose, FBC, Na^+, Ca^{2+}, Mg^{2+}, K^+, urea, creatinine, clotting, X-match, blood culture.
— Antibiotics: Ceftriaxone (80 mg/Kg) or if < 1m, cefotaxime (50 mg/Kg).
— Correct shock if present: **Fluid bolus: 20ml/Kg, 5–10 min, if there are clear signs of under-perfusion + early inotropes + metabolic corrections (see above).**
— Dexamethasone
— Neurointensive care as per protocol (page 130).
— Treat seizures as per protocol (page 125).
— Call anaesthetists and PICU early!

<u>Prophylaxis of household contacts:</u> **Page 224.**

— Inform the Public Health Department.
— Ciprofloxacin one dose:
<5 y: 30 mg/Kg (max 125 mg); 5–12 y: 250 mg;
>12 y: 500 mg.

Confirming the diagnosis:

Lumbar puncture: not if in shock or RICP.
To do ONLY if there are signs of meningitis <u>AND NO</u> typical rash <u>AND NO</u> contraindications (page 124). Waiting for an LP should not delay antibiotics.
Other tests: Blood cultures, throat swab, whole blood (EDTA) for PCR, rapid latex antigen test.

Vaccines:

— 1999 polysaccharide conjugate vaccine against serogroup C: Highly effective; disappearance of serogroup C disease.
— 2010 quadrivalent (serogroup A, C, W135, Y) polysaccharide conjugate vaccine for anyone aged 2–55 y.
— 2013: Multicomponent recombinant protein vaccine for serogroup B from 2m of age. Prior to this, the difficulty of creating a B vaccine had been that the capsular polysaccharide on B meningococci was too similar to human cells to be a useful vaccine target.

NECROTISING FASCIITIS

Principles & Practice of Pediatric Infectious Diseases,
3rd ed., Elsevier, 2008.
Hashan S. *Necrotising fasciitis. BMJ,* 2005, 330: 830–833.
Reviewed by Simon Nadel and Ruchi Sinha, 2013

Necrotising fasciitis is a fulminating disease leading to rapidly spreading necrosis of fascia subcutaneous tissue sometimes involving muscle and skin. If untreated it leads to shock with multiorgan failure and death. Even with surgery mortality is 20–40%.

Causes:

— Not identifiable in some cases.
— History of trauma, injury, burns, minor cuts, insect bites.
— Pre-existing susceptibility to infection: varicella, vascular disease, diabetes, immunosuppression, drug abusers, chronic renal failure. Beware of a chicken pox vesicle around which the skin is inflamed.
— Usually caused by *Group A β haemolytic Streptococcus* which can grow from cultures of wounds and surgically debrided tissues. May be polymicrobial.

Signs:

— Most often on extremities, perineum, truncal areas.
— Erythema, pain, swelling over the infected area.
— Severe pain disproportionate to local findings.

— Induration and oedema.
— Rapidly progressing infection.
— Signs of severe systemic toxicity, shock (pages 9–21, 47).

<u>Treatment:</u> This is a surgical emergency!

— Supportive therapy for multiorgan failure and shock (page 47).
— Antibiotics to start immediately: ceftriaxone + clindamycin + gentamicin (until organism is confirmed) (page 232).
— Urgent extensive surgical debridement must not be delayed.
— IVIG 2 g/Kg over 10 h may improve the prognosis and can be given to shocked patients with Staphylococcal or Streptococcal infection.

NEONATAL SEPSIS AND MENINGITIS
Principles & Practice of Pediatric Infectious Diseases,
3rd ed., Elsevier, 2008.
Summary by Claudine De Munter

Early onset bacterial septicaemia: First 7 days, non-focal, fulminant. Often the maternal genital tract is the source; Group B Streptococcus (GBS), *E.coli* are the predominant pathogens.

Late onset: Usually starts focal (urinary tract, pneumonia, bone, joint): *Staphylococcus, GBS, E.coli, Enterococcus, Enterobacter, Klebsiella* are the most common.

Signs:

— Subtle, non-specific.
— Initially, there may be only one sign before rapid deterioration: E.g. initially, the only sign can be <u>repetitive vomiting</u> for a day.
— Other signs: Fever, poor feeding, vomiting, irritability, lethargy, respiratory signs, bradycardia, unexplained tachycardia, diarrhoea, apnoea, jaundice, hyper/hypoglycaemia, hypothermia, abdominal distension, back-arching, bulging fontanelle (meningitis), seizure, hyper/hypoglycaemia, hypothermia, shock (pages 9–21).

Treatment:

Antibiotics must not be delayed by the desire to have a diagnosis: cefotaxime + amoxicillin + gentamicin. Add vancomycin if a bone/joint is involved. Add metronidazole if there are abdominal signs (page 223).

Cultures and tests:

— Cultures must be obtained as soon as possible without delaying administration of antibiotics, with at least blood cultures, urine cultures and CSF cultures if possible. An LP must be obtained if safe (page 124).
— X-ray.
— Ultrasound.

Blood tests are relatively unhelpful:

WCC can be <5000 or >20000 but many patients have a normal WCC. Thrombocytopenia: insensitive, non-specific. CRP increased: sensitivity 50–90%.

FEVER IN ONCOLOGY/IMMUNOCOMPROMISED/ BONE MARROW TRANSPLANT (BMT) PATIENTS

http://source/prdcont/groups/extranet/@clinical/@ guidelines/documents/ppgs/smh_019001.pdf

Reviewed by Leena Karnik, 2014

Febrile neutropenia:

Absolute neutrophil count $<0.5 \times 10^9$/L in oncology cases or $<1.0 \times 10^9$/L in BMT cases <u>AND</u>

— Fever $\geq$38 °C, even if measured just once.

— <u>OR</u> clinical suspicion of sepsis in absence of fever (e.g. unexplained abdominal pain, rigors, compensated or uncompensated hypotensive shock).

Fever in BMT/Oncology/Immunocompromised patient:

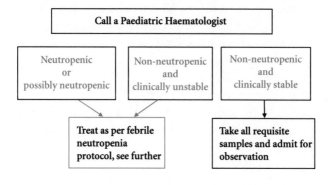

— Immediate assessment and admission to a cubicle (pages 9–21).
— Within the <u>first hour</u> of assessment, it is necessary to have done a full clinical examination + blood cultures + antibiotics.
— As soon as possible, do the other investigations as required.

<u>Initial investigations:</u>

Mark specimens as 'neutropenic'.

— Full clinical examination including looking for mucositis, ulcers, thrush, central venous catheters for exit site/tunnel infections.
— Blood cultures pre-treatment are essential: Culture each lumen of central venous line (discard 3–5 ml, up to 10 ml depending on the size of the child) or do peripheral cultures if there is no central line. A Portacath *in situ* must be accessed and cultures taken unless there is skin or soft tissue infection at the site in which case peripheral access is best.
— Urine M,C&S always.
— Swabs from sites of clinical infection: cultures and viral immunofluorescence (IF) or PCR.
— Stools (if diarrhoea): M,C&S, *Clostridium difficile* toxin, rotavirus or adenovirus antigen, cryptosporidium antigen.
— Sputum: M,C&S as indicated.
— NPA/throat swab: culture, PCR/IF (respiratory viruses).
— Chest X-ray: If there are chest symptoms or signs.

Treatment:

Antibiotics to administer within 1 hour of medical assessment:

Tazocin (piperacillin/tazobactam) IV, 90 mg/Kg, 4 times a day, AND Gentamicin IV, 7 mg/Kg once daily. Check level prior to second dose. See BNF(C) for caution. Add Vancomycin IV, 20 mg/Kg, 3 times a day, OR Teicoplanin if there is a tunnelled line infection, an exit site infection or an endoprostheses infection (10 mg/Kg twice a day for first 3 doses then 10 mg/Kg every 24 h) (page 231).

Things to remember:

— Continue all prophylaxis treatment: Cotrimoxazole, anti-viral and so on.
— Stop the oral chemotherapy the patient may be taking at home.
— Treat hypotensive shock as per guidelines (page 47).
— Use of blood products for supportive care as per guidelines: Transfuse RBC if Hb < 7 g/dl and give platelets if $<20 \times 10^9$/L. Use CMV negative, irradiated blood if special requirements are not known.
— Pain: Supportive care management as per protocol (page 191).
— Mucositis: Treat as per local Oncology Supportive Care guidelines.

SEVERE MALARIA
Lubell Y *et al. Bulletin of WHO*, 2011, 89: 504–512.
Reviewed by Shunmay Yeung, 2011

Suspicion and diagnosis:

Think of malaria in any child even if anti-malarial prophylaxis was taken.

— Fever is <u>almost</u> always present.
— Symptoms may be non-specific: 'Flu-like', vomiting, diarrhoea.
— Deterioration happens very quickly: Cerebral (seizure, coma), DIC, haemolysis, hypoglycaemia, renal failure, pulmonary oedema.

Diagnosis:

— Thick and thin films for microscopy (EDTA blood).
Repeat 3 times if initially negative and diagnosis suspected.
— Rapid antigen screen.

DANGER: <5y: parasite count >5% OR, all ages with parasite count >10%.

Differential diagnosis:

Always look for other possible coexisting infections: viruses, bacteria including typhoid and parasites.
Tests: FBC, blood glucose (BM), blood cultures, blood gases, lactate, CRP, urea, creatinine, electrolytes, liver, X-match, sickle cell status, G6PD status, urine microscopy and culture, throat swab, LP if possible (page 124).

Recognition of severe malaria: **Pages 9–21.**

Malaria will be severe if any of the following is present.

— Depressed GCS.	— Status epilepticus (page 123).
— Increased work of breathing.	— Shock/dehydration (page 47).
— Metabolic acidosis (BD > 8).	— Severe hyperkalaemia (page 109).

Initiate treatment:

— Give IV artesunate 2.4 mg/Kg, slow IV, at 0, 12, 24 hours then daily until oral medication is tolerated.

— OR loading dose IV quinine (2nd choice) 20 mg/Kg (max 1.4 g) in 5–10% dextrose over 4 h then 10 mg/Kg over 4 h, tds, until oral medication is tolerated.

Severe malaria — complications and management:

— Respiratory failure: high flow O_2 15 L/min face mask with reservoir bag or intubation as indicated (pages 9–21, 183).

— Shock (page 47).

— Seizure/coma/RICP (pages 119–130).

— Hypoglycaemia is very frequent (pages 158, 219).

Call PICU and anaesthetists early.

Signs of shock:

Summary (page 47):

— A/B/C management, 2 IV cannulae.
— Monitoring RR, SaO$_2$, HR, BP, CRT, pulses, blood gases.
— Give 10–20 ml/Kg 0.9% saline over 1 hour or faster depending on the BP and other signs (above).
— Elective intubation after 40 ml/Kg if shock persists (pages 47, 183).
— Correct hypoglycaemia, electrolyte abnormalities (pages 107, 158, 219).
— Consider coexisting RICP (page 130).

Signs of coma/seizure:
(tonic-clonic, complex seizures)

Summary (pages 119–123):

— A/B/C management, 2 IV cannulae.
— Monitoring RR, SaO$_2$, HR, BP, CRT, blood gases.
— Check glucose (page 219).
— Follow status epilepticus algorithm (page 123).
— Consider coexisting shock and RICP (pages 47, 130).

RICP:

Summary (page 130):

— 30 degrees, head mid line.
— Elective intubation.
— Good oxygenation (pages 183–187).
— Maintain PaCO$_2$ to 4.5–5.3 KPa.
— Bolus 3% saline (or ready-made 2.7% saline) or mannitol as required (page 218).
— Cautious fluid resuscitation and early use of inotropes to maintain BP high normal (page 217).

OSTEOMYELITIS/SEPTIC ARTHRITIS: URGENT MANAGEMENT
Managing bone and joint infection in children.
Faust S *et al. Arch Dis Child*, 2012, 97(6): 545–553.
Reviewed by Jethro Herberg, 2013

Diagnosis:

OM: Osteomyelitis. SA: Septic arthritis.

— Delayed treatment leads to joint destruction or chronic infection.
— SA: Infection of synovial joints. It is a surgical emergency.
— OM: Haematogenous/contiguous spread/direct inoculation.

Often long bones: femur > tibia > humerus. It can also be multifocal.

— Co-incidence of OM and SA: Common and best distinguished by MRI.

Predisposing factors:

Skin and soft tissue infection/trauma/sickle cell disease/recent respiratory infection/joint pathology (prosthesis, juvenile idiopathic arthritis)/CVL/ immunodeficiency.

Pathogens: **Page 231.**

— Previously healthy children: *Staphylococcus aureus* (44–80%), *Kingella kingae* (14–50% infants <36 m). *Group A Streptococcus, Streptococcus pneumonia, Haemophilus influenzae,* Panton–Valentine Leukocidin (PVL) producing *Staphylococcus aureus* (causing severe infections, often multifocal, pneumonias, recurrent boils).

— Neonates: Group B Streptococcus, *E.coli*, other gram-negatives, fungi. 40% of cases are multifocal.
— Neonates and adolescents: *Gonococcus.*
— If long history of osteoarticular problems: mycobacteria, coxiella, brucella, bartonella, fungi. Other: Metabolic, malignant, rheumatological.
— Sickle cell disease (page 41): *Salmonella* and *Pneumococcus.*

Clinical features:

— Pain of joint/limb and reluctance to move, fever, local redness, hot, soft tissue swelling.
— Deep joint (e.g. hip) SA: Only sign may be decreased range of movement.
— Sickle cell disease (page 41): All of the above may be present in vaso-occlusive crisis mimicking OM.

Differential diagnosis:

Long list including systemic diseases, post infective, NAI/trauma, local issues, metabolic and rheumatological disorders or malignancies.

Management:

Multidisciplinary from admission: Orthopaedics, Paediatrics, Microbiology and Radiology. Haematology in case of sickle cell disease.

— Do not delay referral waiting for scans.
— Septic children with SA or OM: Call surgeons, start antibiotics.

Investigations on admission:

— FBC, CRP, blood cultures, save serum (for differential diagnosis).

74

— Swab throat and other sites, do <u>MRSA swabs</u>.
— X-ray: To check for fracture or foreign body; to monitor treatment response.
— Ultrasound: For joint effusions, soft tissue swelling, periosteal reaction or fluid collection.
— MRI: Investigation of choice, as soon as possible, before surgery. It helps in differentiating between OM and SA.

<u>Septic arthritis:</u>

— If effusion is clinically apparent and seen on US: Urgent joint washout.
— Non-septic children with effusion: Delay antibiotics until after joint washout UNLESS this is expected to take more than 4 hours.
— Send for M,C&S, protein, glucose, molecular studies if indicated.

<u>Osteomyelitis:</u>

— Treatment initiated on clinical signs. Do not delay antibiotics: Start IV antibiotics after blood cultures.
— If no fluid collection: No surgery needed in the acute phase.
— For sickle cell patients, involve haematologists. It may be difficult to distinguish osteonecrosis due to vaso-occlusive crisis from OM.

<u>Antibiotics and ancillary treatments:</u> **Page 231.**

Ceftriaxone IV and clindamycin IV/PO.

— PVL *Staphylococcus aureus*: Add LMW heparin for DVT prophylaxis, IVIG, aggressive surgical debridement. Request PVL typing.
— *Group A Streptococcus*: Add LMW heparin (DVT risk is also high).

— Presence of CVL or known MRSA carriage: Add vancomycin.
— Septic children <3 m: Add amoxicillin until listeria is excluded.
— Reinvestigate all children who are still febrile at 72 hours.

Duration of IV treatment and changing to oral antibiotics:

— Give IV for >2–3 w if <3 m, or multifocal, or severe infection, or immunocompromised, or no organism isolated, or multiresistant organism.
— Change to oral treatment if:
  • the situation is not one of the above
  • <u>AND</u> the patient is afebrile >48 hours
  • <u>AND</u> the patient is clinically improved
  • <u>AND</u> the CRP is less than 20
  • <u>AND</u> the patient can tolerate oral therapy.

CARDIAC – SPECIFIC

SUPRAVENTRICULAR TACHYCARDIA (SVT)
APLS 2012. ERC 2010 guidelines. 2010 American Heart Association guidelines. 2010 International Consensus on Cardiopulmonary Resuscitation and Emergency Cardiovascular Care Science with Treatment Recommendations (COSTR).
Reviewed by David Inwald, Margarita Burmester, 2012

Cause:
Primary: Congenital re-entrant pathways.
Secondary: See below.

Assess: Pages 9–21, 47.
Initial signs can be non-specific signs of an unwell patient or signs of cardiogenic shock if SVT is too prolonged.
— Definition: SVT: HR > 220–300 bpm — regular, no beat-to-beat variability. P waves may or may not be present. QRS usually narrow.
— Differential: Sinus tachycardia: HR <220 in infants, <180 in children + a compatible history or known cause + P waves present and normal + beat-to-beat variability + variable R-R + constant PR.
— Assess ABC, ECG rhythm strip + 12 lead ECG. Consider expert opinion.
— Prepare for cardioversion or adenosine. Is the child in cardiogenic shock? Evaluate A? B? CRT, BP, pulses? Core/toe temperature gap? Gallop rhythm? Liver? Mental state? Blood gas?

— Electrolytes (Mg^{2+}, Ca^{2+} and K^+): Correct to high normal levels (pages 107–110).
— Consider possible aetiologies (below).

Treat possible causes:
Hypoxia, hypovolaemia, hypothermia, hypo/hyperkalaemia/metabolic acidosis, tension pneumothorax, tamponade, cardiac toxins, thromboembolism, trauma.

Indications for intubation
(call PICU): Pages 183, 187

— Cardiac failure with acidosis.
— Impending cardio-respiratory collapse.

Management following intubation
(call PICU, cardiologists):

— Correct shock and acidosis: 10ml/Kg boluses 0.9% saline, cautiously.
— Consider bicarbonate. Consider inotropic support (but beware, inotropes may precipitate further dysrhythmias) (pages 109, 217).
— Call cardiologists: Consider amiodarone 5 mg/Kg IV over 20–60 min (page 218). If resistant, ECMO may be needed.

Supraventricular Tachycardia (SVT)

Differential diagnosis with ECG; Tachycardia with pulse present:

— Wide QRS > 0.08sec: ventricular tachycardia; look at a 'wide complex tachycardia' protocol.
— Narrow QRS < 0.08 sec: sinus tachycardia or SVT.

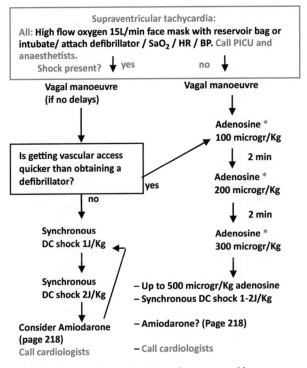

Supraventricular tachycardia:
All: High flow oxygen 15L/min face mask with reservoir bag or intubate/ attach defibrillator / SaO₂ / HR / BP. Call PICU and anaesthetists.
Shock present? ↓ yes   no ↓

Vagal manoeuvre (if no delays)   **Vagal manoeuvre**

Adenosine * 100 microgr/Kg
↓ 2 min
Is getting vascular access quicker than obtaining a defibrillator?   **Adenosine * 200 microgr/Kg**
yes
no ↓   ↓ 2 min
Synchronous DC shock 1J/Kg   **Adenosine * 300 microgr/Kg**

Synchronous DC shock 2J/Kg   – Up to 500 microgr/Kg adenosine
– Synchronous DC shock 1-2J/Kg

Consider Amiodarone (page 218)   – Amiodarone? (Page 218)
Call cardiologists
– Call cardiologists

* Adenosine needs to be administered as a very rapid bolus +10 ml 0.9% saline

If the patient is conscious, defibrillation will require the presence of an anaesthetist for sedation or tracheal intubation. In case of cardiac failure, the patient is likely to need ventilatory support: CPAP or tracheal intubation. Electrolyte abnormalities (mainly K^+, Ca^{2+}, Mg^{2+}) and low BM need correction to high normal levels to optimise cardiac function (pages 107–110, 219).

DUCT-DEPENDENT CONGENITAL
HEART DISEASE

http://www.neonatal.org.uk/documents/1457.pdf.
London Kent Surrey & Sussex Duct-Dependent
Congenital Heart Disease; Review 2008.
Shekerdemian, P. *Arch Dis Child Fetal Neonatal Ed*,
2001, 84: F141–F145.
Reviewed by Margarita Burmester, 2012

Presentation:

— First few days–months of life: Pages 9–21, 47.
— Difficulty feeding, breathlessness, increasing cyanosis.
— Possibly in heart failure: Tachycardia, tachypnoea, hepatomegaly.
— A murmur may or may not be audible.
— Cardiogenic shock: Grey appearance, weak/absent peripheral pulses, severe metabolic acidosis, leading to multiorgan failure.

Types of duct-dependent lesions:

— Ductus maintains systemic circulation: Coarctation of the aorta, critical aortic stenosis, hypoplastic left heart.
— Ductus maintains pulmonary circulation: Pulmonary atresia (PA), critical pulmonary stenosis, tricuspid atresia (TA), Tetralogy of Fallot.
— Ductus maintains mix of blood of systemic and pulmonary circulations: Transposition of great arteries.

Differential diagnosis:

Sepsis, metabolic disorder, persistent pulmonary hypertension of the newborn (PPHN), primary pulmonary disease, total anomalous pulmonary venous return (TAPVD).

Assessment and treatment:

— Four limb BP, pre- and post-ductal SaO_2, ECG, hyperoxia test.
— Intubate if required: If in shock or when prostaglandin is started at >10 nanogr/Kg/min.
— Give O_2 to keep SaO_2 80–85% (higher SaO_2 increases the risk of duct closure; lower SaO_2 causes hypoxia).
— Shock: 0.9% saline 10 ml/Kg (max 30 ml/Kg). Start dopamine if shock persists. Check BM regularly. Correct hypoglycaemia. Pages 217, 219.
— Commence IV antibiotics.
— Assess and correct acidosis: Page 109.
— Transfer to a cardiac unit.

Drug choices and errors:

— <u>Do not use</u> prostacyclin (epoprostenol, flolan). They are used for PPHN.
— Drug of choice: dinoprostone (= Prostin, PGE2). Some hospitals use alprostadil (PGE1) 10–100 nanogr/Kg/min.

Transfer to a cardiac unit:

Intubate if shock or high risks of apnoea with prostaglandin (if doses PGE_2>10 nanogr/Kg/min): Page 183.

Duct-Dependent Congenital Heart Disease

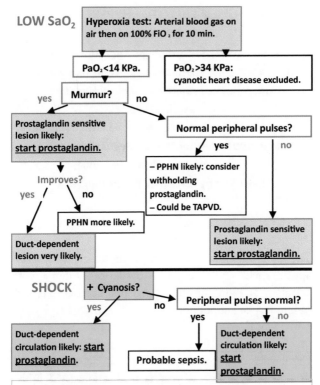

LOW SaO₂ — Hyperoxia test: Arterial blood gas on air then on 100% FiO₂ for 10 min.

PaO₂ <14 KPa.

PaO₂ >34 KPa: cyanotic heart disease excluded.

Murmur? — yes / no

yes → Prostaglandin sensitive lesion likely: **start prostaglandin.**

no → **Normal peripheral pulses?** — yes / no

yes → − PPHN likely: consider withholding prostaglandin. − Could be TAPVD.

no → Prostaglandin sensitive lesion likely: **start prostaglandin.**

Improves? — yes / no

yes → Duct-dependent lesion very likely.

no → PPHN more likely.

SHOCK — + Cyanosis? — yes / no

yes → Duct-dependent circulation likely: **start prostaglandin.**

no → **Peripheral pulses normal?** — yes / no

yes → Probable sepsis.

no → Duct-dependent circulation likely: **start prostaglandin.**

Prostaglandin infusion: INOPROSTONE (PGE2).
Low dose: 3–10 nanogr/Kg/min if patient is not in shock & stable.
High dose starting at 5 increasing up to 50 nanogr/Kg/min if in shock.
Infusion of Dinoprostone (1mg/ml): 0.1ml x weight in Kg = ml of dinoprostone to be drawn up (= 100 microgr x weight in Kg). Make up to 33ml of 0.9% saline or dextrose. 0.1ml/h = 5 nanogr/Kg/min. Adverse effects: apnoea, bradycardia, hypotension, fever, hypoglycaemia.
Monitoring of vital signs is essential. Bag/mask for ventilation must be ready before starting PGE₂. Inotropes and resuscitation fluids should also be available. **Pages 9–21, 47, 216, 217.**

TETRALOGY OF FALLOT — HYPERCYANOTIC SPELLS

Starship Paediatric Cardiology, Auckland. Reviewed 2010; www.adhb.govt.nz/starshipclinicalguidelines. Park, MK. The *Pediatric Cardiology Handbook*, Mosby, 2003. Chang AC, *Pediatric Cardiac Intensive Care*, Williams & Wilkins, 1998. Lieh-Lai M *et al.*, *Pediatric Acute Care*, 2nd ed., Williams & Wilkins, 2001. Reviewed by Margarita Burmester, 2012

Background:

The 'TET Spell', 'hypoxic spell', 'cyanotic spell', 'hypercyanotic spell' or 'paroxysmal dyspnoea': Infants with Tetralogy of Fallot, or other congenital heart defects with pulmonary or subpulmonary stenosis and VSD at any age.

Common precipitants:

Crying, defecation, feeding, waking from naps, fever, dehydration, tachypnoea, tachycardia, medications (ACE inhibitors). Common in children who are iron deficient.

Signs and symptoms:

Uncontrollable crying/panic, hyperpnoea, deepening of cyanosis, decreased intensity of heart murmur, limpness, convulsions and, rarely, death.

Hypercyanotic spells need to be recognised quickly and effectively to prevent the development of complications from prolonged hypoxia. Many episodes are self-limiting.

Pathophysiology:

Imbalance between pulmonary and systemic vascular resistance favouring decreased pulmonary flow and increased right-to-left shunting. Hypoxaemia, metabolic acidosis, hyperpnoea, increased systemic venous return, catecholamines and pulmonary vasoconstriction are all thought to be involved in a self-perpetuating cycle. Infundibular spasm is not always present.

Management:

— Knee-to-chest/squatting: Place the child in the knees-to-chest position either lying supine or over the parent's shoulder.
— Oxygen (100%) administered usually has minimal effect.

Keep child calm with parent. Knee-to-chest position. Give O_2 if tolerated.

Cyanosis persists? Start by calming the child.

Indicators of
improved pulmonary
blood flow:
– Decreased cyanosis.
– Louder murmur.

Morphine 0.1 mg/Kg, SC/IM (not IV: apnoea),
OR Buccal midazolam 200–300 microgr/Kg
(max 5mg).

Cyanosis (spell) persists?

no   yes

Correct any
underlying cause
which may
exacerbate episode:
cardiac arrhythmia,
hypothermia,
hypoglycaemia,
anaemia,
hypovolaemia.

M

– Continuous ECG,
– SaO_2, BP monitoring,
– IV line,
– Preload 10–20 ml/Kg IV 0.9% saline,
– Call for expert consultation.

yes

– Observe, keep calm.
– Give oxygen if needed.
– Consider expert opinion.
– Do not send home even
  if crisis is short self-limiting.

– Call PICU.
– Esmolol
0.5 mg/Kg IV over 1 min then
0.05–0.5 mg/Kg/min IV infusion.
– OR propanolol
0.15–0.25 mg/Kg IV.
Repeat once after 15 min.

– Monitoring SaO_2, HR, BP.
– Propanolol 0.5 mg/Kg/dose PO
tds (gradually increase to 1.0–1.5mg/
Kg/dose, tds).
Risks: low BP, hypoglycaemia.

– Metaraminol:
0.01mg/Kg IV bolus than,
infusion 0.1–1 microgr/Kg/min.
or SC/IM 0.1 mg/Kg.
– OR phenylephrine:
IV 5–20 microgr/Kg dose (slowly).
Infusion 0.1–0.5 microgr/Kg/min.

Consider early surgery.

Sodium bicarbonate 1mmol/Kg IV, page 109.
Consider blood transfusion.

Urgent surgery required.
Consider ventilation (use ketamine 1–3mg/Kg), pages 183–187.

MYOCARDITIS: WHEN TO THINK OF IT AND MANAGEMENT OF IT

Paediatric Cardiology, 3rd ed., Anshan, 2010.

Reviewed by Claudine De Munter, Margarita Burmester

Causes:

Infectious: Enterovirus (Coxsackie B), adenovirus, parvovirus B19, CMV, Hep C, HSV, HIV. *Mycobacteria, Streptococcus, Mycoplasma pneumoniae,* syphilis, fungal. Chagas disease (most common cause worldwide).

Immune mediated: Kawasaki disease, page 54.

Toxins: Cocaine.

Signs:

Underdiagnosed; signs are often unspecific or mild.

— May have prodromal symptoms of viraemia: fever, myalgia, coryzal, vomiting, diarrhoea, abdominal pain.

— Cardiomegaly on chest X-ray is the most important clinical sign.

— Neonates and infants: Congestive heart failure may appear acutely; tachycardia, gallop rhythm, tachypnoea.

— Older children: May have mild signs.

— Haemodynamic collapse or sudden death can occur in all groups.

— ECG changes: Any or all of: Low QRS voltage, ST-T changes, prolonged QT interval, arrhythmia including premature contractions.

Prognosis:

Generally this is a fully reversible disease.
— If presenting with cardiac failure most improve within months.
— If severe, ECMO is often needed. Heart transplantation is rarely required.

Diagnosis:
There must be a high index of suspicion of myocarditis in any of these conditions alone or associated:

— Presence of ECG changes, even if asymptomatic.
— Palpitations or syncope (symptomatic ECG changes).
— Sudden infant death: Page 206.
— Haemodynamic instability with prodromal signs of viraemia. This leads to a differential diagnosis with other forms of shock: sepsis, toxic…: Page 47.
— Congestive heart failure.

Tests that may help:

— PCR for viruses.
— Blood gas including pH, base deficit, lactate, electrolytes.
— Troponin I: High specificity, sensitivity 34%. CK, CK-MB are less sensitive.
— Chest X-ray: May be normal but usually shows a large heart ± pulmonary oedema.
— Echocardiography: Cardiac chamber enlargement and impaired left ventricular function.

Thinking of myocarditis in the presence of haemodynamic shock:

Start management for haemodynamic shock: **Page 47.**

Oxygen, fluid boluses, electrolyte and BM corrections, vascular access, inotropes (central IV adrenaline).
Early intubation: See below.
Blood tests as above.
ECG. Chest X-ray.
Antibiotics: Page 228.

Think of myocarditis as a probable cause of shock (page 47) and call a cardiologist:

— If troponin I levels are high.
— If the patient does not improve; lactate level rises despite treatment for shock, liver size increases with fluid boluses and/or pulmonary oedema develops rapidly and/or heart increases in size on X-ray.

Intubation: **Pages 183–187.**

If myocarditis is considered a high risk, choosing the wrong induction agent may cause rapid loss of cardiac output and precipitate death:
— Thiopentone and fentanyl MUST NOT be given as induction agents in shock in general and particularly in the presence of myocarditis.

— Ketamine is the drug of choice with a paralysing agent.
— When possible, prior to intubation it is best to optimise the cardiac function with inotropes and by correcting electrolyte derangements (low Ca^{2+}, low K^+) (pages 47, 107, 217).

FLUIDS/ABDOMINAL/ELECTROLYTES

FLUID MAINTENANCE
APLS 2012.
Updated by David Inwald, 2013

Neonates: 150 ml/Kg/day.
Infants 1–12 m: 100 ml/Kg/day.
Up to 10 Kg: 100 mls/Kg/day.
10–20 Kg: Add to previous another 50 mls/Kg/day for all additional Kg above 10 Kg.
20–30 Kg: Add to previous another 20 mls/Kg/day for all additional Kg above 20 Kg.
>50 Kg: 2–2.5 litres per day.

Prescription of fluids should also consider:

— Hydration status: Page 100.
— Ongoing losses, diarrhoea, stoma losses, vomiting…
— Risks of cerebral oedema: Meningitis, traumatic brain injury, DKA, hypoxic ischaemic encephalopathy: Pages 119, 130, 147, 165.
— Metabolic disorders, hyperinsulinism: Pages 151, 158.
— Increased insensible losses.
— Risk of SIADH: Meningitis, pneumonia, bronchiolitis, post-operative.

Type of fluids and volume:

— Enteral fluids if possible even if dehydrated: Pages 100, 217.

— IV fluids in presence of shock or if enteral feeds are not tolerated/not indicated (vomiting/decreased GCS).

Standard fluid:

— Sodium chloride 0.9% + glucose 5% + 10 or 20 mmol KCl per 500 ml bag.
— Sodium chloride 0.45% + glucose 5% + 10 or 20 mmol KCl per 500 ml bag.

Take into account:

— If serum K^+ is elevated: Omit potassium.
— If serum Na^+ is low: Think of excess Na^+ losses or excess water. SIADH is common.

Fluid restriction:

— Meningitis, cerebral oedema: Restrict to 60% of maintenance: Page 130.
— Post-operatively: Restrict to 60% maintenance on day 1, 80% maintenance on day 2, give 100% maintenance on day 3.

Increased requirements:

High insensible losses: pyrexia, sweating, hypermetabolic states (burns, radiant heaters, phototherapy etc...).

<u>Monitoring:</u>

— Regular weighing: This is the most accurate way of assessing hydration in patients who do not have capilliary leak (e.g. sepsis).

— If on IV fluids: Check electrolytes at least once daily. May need checking 4–6 hrly (i.e. DKA, sepsis, renal failure: Pages 47, 143, 147).

— Be prepared to change fluid prescription as frequently as necessary.

VOMITING AND DEHYDRATION CRITERIA
Reviewed by Michael Coren, 2013

Differential diagnosis of vomiting: Non-specific symptoms

— Gastroenteritis: most common cause.
— Consider other causes when vomiting is present on its own or persists isolated for more than 2 d. Some causes need urgent treatment.
— UTI, acute abdomen (page 112), other abdominal causes (hepatitis…), pneumonia, otitis media, DKA (page 147), shock, sepsis (page 47), myocarditis (page 89), toxic shock (page 57), meningoencephalitis (page 126), RICP (page 130), metabolic disorder (page 155), medications, poisons, allergies (pages 50, 176).

Vomiting children who are at risk:

— If comorbidities are present.
— If less than 6 m.
— If feeding and growth problems.

Managing the vomiting patient:

— Identify the cause and treat it!!
— In gastroenteritis, ondansetron can reduce vomiting (pages 101, 219).
— Food and fluid intake may need to be modified, stopped (e.g. in case of a possible surgical cause) or temporarily given nasogastrically or nasojejunally.

Dehydration Criteria

	MILD	MODERATE	SEVERE
Weight loss	3–5%	6–9%	>10%
Appearance	Normal	Thirsty, lethargic, irritable	Limp, sweaty
Skin turgor	Laxer	Pinch retracts slowly	Very slow
Eyes	Normal	Sunken	Very sunken
Mucosae	Moist	Dry	Very dry
Urine flow	lightly reduced	<1ml/Kg/h	Oliguria
Extremities	Warm	Cool	Cool, mottled
CRT	<2s	>3s	>3s

GASTROENTERITIS
Reviewed by Michael Coren, 2013

Diarrhoeal disease ± nausea, vomiting, fever, abdominal pain.

Differential diagnosis:

— If vomiting ± some diarrhoea: acute abdomen? UTI? DKA? (Pages 112, 147.)
— If child is 'toxic-looking': Could be sepsis, haemodynamic shock (page 47).
— If bloody diarrhoea: Bacterial infection, haemolytic uraemic syndrome, colitis, intussusception?
— If bile-stained vomiting: Small bowel obstruction? Sepsis?
— If severe abdominal pain: Acute abdomen, DKA, renal tract disorder?

Calculation of fluid requirements: **Pages 95, 219.**

Normal maintenance: <10 Kg: 100 ml/Kg; 10–20 Kg: 1000 + 50 ml per kilo above 10; >20 Kg: 1500 + 20 ml per kilo above 20. >50 Kg: 2–2.5 L/day.

Replacement for dehydration: % dehydration × weight (Kg) × 10 = fluid deficit in ml. Add to maintenance volume as calculated above.

Also remember the ongoing losses if diarrhoea or vomiting continue.

Management:

Take a full history and do a complete examination + weigh the child correctly and daily.

Do a urine analysis including dipstix.

— ≥10% dehydrated or signs of shock or unconscious:
  IV access, blood tests, 20 ml/Kg 0.9% saline, consider other diagnosis.

— 6–9% dehydrated:
  Oral rehydration solution (Diorylate/Electrolade) 100 ml/Kg over 4 h + replace ongoing losses (spoon or syringe).
  If the child tolerates oral rehydration: continue over 4–6 h.
  If vomiting <u>and</u> diagnosis is correct: Ondansetron as a stat dose + change to NG oral rehydration solution given continuously over 20 h. Call a specialist.
  If vomiting continues: Blood tests + start IV fluids (maintenance + losses 0.9% saline and 5% dextrose).

— Once rehydrated and not vomiting:
  Resume breast feeding, formula, milk, recommended foods and continue to replace ongoing losses with oral rehydration solution. Lactose containing foods can be resumed.

— 3–5% dehydrated:
  Oral rehydration solution (Diorylate/Electrolade) at 50 ml/Kg over 4 h + replace ongoing losses (spoon or syringe).

— ≤ 3% dehydrated:
  Continue child's age-appropriate diet oral rehydration solution to replace stool losses, or give more than usual dietary fluids.

Hypernatraemia: Page 103. Defined as Na^+ >150. Use 0.9% saline and 5% dextrose. Replace deficit slowly to obtain a Na^+ drop of <0.5 mmol/L/h.

HYPERNATRAEMIA
Reviewed by Jane Deal, 2013

Definition:

Serum sodium >150 mmol/L.

Differential diagnosis:

Dehydration versus salt poisoning.

It is vital to obtain information and investigations on presentation or the diagnosis will be impossible to make and important evidence may be not be present.

History:

Weight loss pre-admission, polyuria, polydipsia, vomiting, diarrhoea, feeding (include obtaining samples of bottled milk), neonatal history, medication history.

Mandatory clinical measurements:

Weight on admission and daily, fractional excretion of Na^+ on admission and daily, fluid balance 4 hrly and daily.

Causes:

— Salt poisoning: Deliberate or accidental or hyperaldosteronism.
— Water deficit (dehydration): Inadequate fluid intake, breast-fed babies, neurological impairment, anorexia,

diarrhoea and vomiting (pages 99–101), burns (page 169), nephrogenic or central diabetes insipidus.

Investigations:

— To do immediately once hypernatraemia is diagnosed.
— Place a urine catheter to obtain urine sample at presentation and to monitor subsequent urine output.
— <u>Blood tests</u>: Na^+, K^+, chloride, bicarbonate, urea, creatinine, osmolality, FBC, plasma renin, aldosterone, random cortisol, random glucose.
— <u>Urine</u>: Na^+, K^+, chloride, bicarbonate, urea, creatinine, osmolality, dipstix.

Treatment:

— Insert an IV line.

<u>Volume and rate of fluid:</u>

Fluid requirements per day = water deficit per day + maintenance fluids per day (page 101).
Divided by 24 = hrly fluids rate to adjust as often as needed depending on fluid balance and serum Na^+ level.
— Volume:
Water deficit = 4 ml/Kg for each 1 mmol/L serum Na^+ <u>over</u> 145 mmol/L.
Maintenance fluids: page 95.
— Fluid: Normal (0.9%) saline initially.

<u>Adjustments:</u>

— Adjust fluid rate depending on fluid balance and Na^+ levels.

  Reduce serum sodium at a rate ≤0.5 mmol/L/h and a maximum drop of 15 mmol/d. **Rapid drop in Na^+ level may cause central pontine myelinolysis.**

— Monitoring for adjustments: Frequent (at least 4 hrly) assessments of fluid balance and serum Na^+ must be done until the serum Na^+ is within the normal range.

Changing the rate of fluid at which the water deficit is replaced:

— If the rate of fall of the serum sodium is too fast, decrease the rate of fluid being given. The 4 hrly measurements of Na^+ will allow you to do this adjustment on a 4 hrly basis if necessary.

— If the rate of fall of serum sodium is too slow, either increase the rate of fluids being given or change the IV fluid to 0.45% saline. The 4 hrly measurements of Na^+ will allow you to do this adjustment on a 4 hrly basis if necessary.

Example:

32 Kg child with serum Na^+ 165 mmol/L.

Maintenance fluids $= (10\,Kg \times 100) + (10\,Kg \times 50)$
$\qquad\qquad\qquad\quad + (12\,Kg \times 20)$
$\qquad\qquad\quad = 1000mls + 500mls + 240mls$
$\qquad\qquad\quad = 1740 \text{ ml}/24\,h$

Water deficit
$$= 4 \times 32 \times (165{-}145)$$
$$= 4 \times 32 \times 20$$
$$= 2560\,\text{ml}/24\,\text{h}$$

Maintenance + deficit
$$= 2560 + 1740\ \text{mls} = 4300\ \text{ml/day} = 179\ \text{ml/h.}$$

ACUTE ELECTROLYTE CORRECTIONS: HCO_3^-, NA^+, K^+, CA^{2+}, MG^{2+}

Updated by Penny Fletcher, Ruchi Sinha, Claudine De Munter, Jane Deal, 2013

KCl for hypokalaemia (<3.5 mmol/L):

Major signs:

Cardiac arrhythmias, muscle weakness, hypotension, ileus.

Dose:

0.2–1 mmol/Kg, at a rate of 0.2 mmol/Kg/h. A higher rate of 0.5 mmol/Kg/h requires a central IV/IO access and BP, ECG monitoring.

— IV peripheral correction OVER 2 HOURS; Use a 500 ml bag of 5% glucose or 0.9% saline. Add KCL, 20 mmol, to obtain a concentration of KCL 40 mmol/l. Give 10 ml/Kg (OVER 2 HOURS). This will give 0.4mmol/Kg of K^+ OVER 2 HOURS.
— IV centrally including IO: Use bags with high concentration of KCL at 0.4 mmol/ml (= 40 mmol/100 ml). Give KCL 0.2–1 mmol/Kg, at a maximum rate of 0.5 mmol/Kg/h and up to 40 mmol/h.

NaCl for hyponatraemia (<135 mmol/L; Danger if <125 mmol/L):

References:

Au, AK *et al.*, *J Pediatr*, 2008, 152(1): 33–38.
Gross, P, *Kidney Int*, 2001, 60(6): 2417–2427.

Knowing the underlying cause is essential: Hyponatraemia can be associated with hyper/normo/hypovolaemia.

Major signs:

Seizure, confusion, coma, brain stem herniation appear with a rapid fall of Na^+ level or when Na^+ <125 mmol/L.

Treatment:

— <u>Symptomatic patients:</u> Use 3% saline (or 2.7% saline pre-made bags if available), 3 ml/Kg bolus, repeated until symptoms stop. Usually this corresponds to a rise of Na^+ of 4–6 mmol/L. See page 218 on how to prepare 3% saline.
— <u>If asymptomatic:</u> To increase Na^+ level to 125 mmol/L, give IV Na^+mmol = $(125 - $ serum $Na^+) \times 0.3 \times$ weight (Kg), over 30–60 min.
— <u>If IV peripherally:</u> Use concentrations of 1.8% saline (300 mmol/L of NaCl) (page 217).
— A rapid rise of Na^+ above 125 mmol/L can cause demyelination. So, if the patient is asymptomatic and/or Na^+>125 mmol/L, Na^+ rise must be <8 mmol/L/day.
— Also treat volume changes: Give volume if there is hypovol-aemia or fluid restrict/diuretics if there is hypervolaemia.

Hypomagnesaemia ($Mg^{2+} < 0.75$ mmol/L):

Major signs:

Muscle weakness, arrhythmias, tetany, seizure.
Often associated with hypokalaemia or hypocalcaemia.
Give 0.2 mmol/Kg over 30 min. Use 50% $MgSO_4$ IV centrally/IO or dilute 5 times in 0.9% saline if a peripheral IV line is used. The 10% solution can be used neat. Beware of dropping BP as a direct effect of Mg^{2+}.

Metabolic acidosis requiring bicarbonate:

— Volume (ml) to give IV of 8.4% $NaHCO_3^-$ to correct the deficit:
   $0.3 \times$ weight (in Kg) $\times$ base deficit/2, over 20 min.
— Neonates: Use 4.2% $NaHCO_3^-$: $0.3 \times$ weight (in Kg) $\times$ base deficit, IV, over 1h.
— 1–2 mmol/Kg, IV over 1 h is an alternative dosage.
— Danger of extravasation injuries and hypernatraemia.
— Not to use in DKA or cardiac arrest unless discussed with intensivists.

Hyperkalaemia >5.5 mmol/L (premature: >6.5 mmol/L):

Reference:

Pediatric hyperkalemia: treatment and management: Michael Verive, 2011. Reviewed by Jane Deal, 2013.

Major symptoms:

Arrhythmias when severe; ECG shows peaked T waves, wide QRS, sine pattern wave form.

Treatment:

1. Adequate volume expansion: 10–20 ml/Kg 0.9% saline.
2. Stabilising myocardium: calcium gluconate 10% 0.1 mmol/Kg over 5–10 min. (Beware of extravasations and arrythmias).
3. Intracellular K^+ shift:
— Sodium bicarbonate 1–2 mmol/Kg, IV over 15–60 min (not with calcium).
— Insulin/dextrose: Insulin 0.1 units/Kg + glucose 0.5g/Kg (= 5 ml/Kg of 10% dextrose), over 30 min–2h. Monitor sugar level (may drop!).
— Salbutamol nebuliser, 2.5 mg or 5 mg (page 215).
— Salbutamol bolus IV. Doses page 216.
4. Enhance body elimination: Calcium resonium powder PO/PR. To use as second stage. PO 125–250 mg/Kg (max 15 g), 6–8 hrly, with water. PR 125–250 mg/Kg in 1–3 mL/Kg of methylcellulose solution or water, 3–4 hrly. Irrigate colon after 6–12 hours to remove resin.
— Furosemide IV 0.5–1 mg/Kg.
— Haemodialysis/haemofiltration.

Hypocalcaemia with ionised calcium <1 mmol/L:

Causes:

Vitamin D deficiency, hypoparathyroidism, low Ca^{++} intake, low Mg^{++}, pseudohypoparathyroidism, familial hypercalcyuric hypocalcaemia.

Major symptoms:

Seizures, cramps, arrhythmias.

Treatment:

— IV if symptomatic (oral if asymptomatic: see BNF for doses).

  IV $CaCl_2$ 0.1 mmol/Kg or IV Calcium gluconate 10% 0.1mmol/Kg.

  Both over 5–10 min (max rate of 0.045 mmol/Kg/h).

— If <u>IV peripheral:</u> Calcium gluconate 10% (= 0.225 mmol Ca^{++}/ml), dilute 5 times.

— If <u>IV central:</u> Calcium gluconate is preferable or use calcium chloride 14.7% (=1 mmol Ca^{++}/ml). Beware of extravasation or precipitations if wrongly administered with phosphate or bicarbonate or IV ceftriaxone.

ABDOMINAL SURGICAL EMERGENCIES —
Bowel Obstruction or Necrosis:
How to Diagnose and What to do Before Surgical Referral.
Reviewed By Shamshad Syed, Munther Haddad, 2012

<u>Abnormal signs and symptoms:</u> **Pages 9–21.**

— Temperature if infection is present or peritonitis.
— Vomiting: Projectile? Yellow or green? Bilious vomiting is an emergency.
— Off feeds?
— Stools: No stools? No gas? Bloody? Projectile? Mucous?
— Unusual cries, irritability or lethargy: Pain? Discomfort? Shock and sepsis?
— Abdominal distension: usually present, though <u>not always</u> present.

<u>Examination and clinical evaluation in all cases:</u>

— Monitor all vital signs: SaO_2, RR, BP. Blood gas. Feel pulses, measure CRT. Increased work of breathing? Under-ventilating (pain)? RR and HR can be higher than expected for age and temperature. BP can be high (pain, agitation), normal, low (decompensated shock).
— Increased gastric aspirates: Gastric aspirates must be measured via an NG tube.

Normal NG aspirates: Volume should be lower than the equivalent of 4 hours' worth of feed and should look like milk or digested milk.

Abnormal NG aspirates: Green/bilious/volumes above 4 hours' worth of feed.

— Abdomen distended? Discoloured? Tender? Mass? Peritonitis?
— Rebound pain on examination (peritoneal irritation) is difficult to assess.
— Sounds: Increased (acute obstruction), absent (peritonitis/perforation).

Beware of:

— Patients immunocompromised or with nephrotic syndrome: Perforations can occur with no pain, minimal distension. There will be vomiting and/or increased gastric aspirates and absent bowel sounds.
— Pneumonia in the lower lobes can be responsible for acute abdominal pain ± other abdominal signs. Tonsillitis can present with abdominal pain.
— Gynaecological/obstetrical issues in teenagers and urinary infections may present with abdominal pain.

Pre-surgical initial management in all cases:

1. Resuscitation as required (page 47).
2. Stop feeds. IV fluid maintenance.
3. Nasogastric tube on free drainage. Nil by mouth.
4. Abdominal X-ray.

5. Ultrasound of abdomen useful in some situations: Intussusception, malrotation, pyloric stenosis, abscess, free fluid.
6. Investigations: Blood gas, glucose, lactate, FBC, U&E, amylase, liver enzymes, bilirubin, CRP, X-match, clotting, urine culture.
7. Antibiotics: Start co-amoxiclav + metronidazole + gentamicin.
8. Call surgeons early.

Neonate –2 months:

Bilious vomiting: 70% cases are surgical, others are likely to be sepsis!

— Abdomen distended: Distal obstruction likely.
— Abdomen flat or scaphoid: Proximal obstruction more likely.
— Malrotation, volvulus and enterocolitis: **Fatal outcomes if not dealt with early. Can present at any age. Do an urgent limited upper GI contrast study. Abdominal tenderness with malrotation is an emergency (urgent laparotomy). Management as above.**
— Volvulus: **Management as above. Urgent surgery required.**
— Necrotising enterocolitis: **Management as above. If early, it may not require surgery.**
— Enterocolitis secondary to Hirschsprung's disease: **Management as above and urgent decompression of bowel (rectal wash out or stoma) required.**

<u>Non-bilious projectile vomit:</u> Pyloric stenosis? **Alkalosis** may be present. Management as above. Surgery required but not urgent.

Infant:

— Intussusception: It is common between 2 m to 2 y. Classic presentation is of a healthy baby who becomes disinterested in feed, crying in sudden episodes that spontaneously stop then the baby remains calm, looking unhappy. <u>Stools:</u> Normal or loose or 'redcurrant jelly' (positive in 50% of cases, usually late). Abdominal distension may be a late presentation. Management as above.
— Malrotation or volvulus: **As above.**
— Incarcerated hernia **more commonly inguinal. May cause intestinal obstruction. Management as above.**
— Meckel's band **can cause bowel obstruction. More than 50% present with painless severe rectal bleeding requiring blood transfusion.**

Children with abdominal pain:

Pre-school age is the most difficult age for diagnosis. Check throat and chest for tonsillitis and pneumonia that are common causes of abdominal pain.

— Malrotation **can present at any age. Management as above.**

— Appendicitis: **Generalised tenderness, high tempera-ture ± signs of peritonitis (perforated appendicitis). Management as above.**
— **If there is a history of previous surgery,** obstruction due to adhesions **is likely.**

NEUROLOGY: GENERAL/SEPSIS RELATED

DECREASED CONSCIOUS LEVEL:
GCS <15 OR AVPU <A
CATS (Children Acute Transport Service) 2011.
The Paediatric A&E Research Group 2008.
Summary by Claudine De Munter

Differential diagnosis:

Meningoencephalopathy (page 126), space occupying lesion, status epilepticus (page 123), post-convulsive state, shock including sepsis (page 47), respiratory failure, hypertension (page 141, poisoning (page 176), trauma (including NAI, page 201), metabolic/endocrine/electrolyte (pages 107, 151) abnormality.

Initial management:

— Give O_2 (mask + reservoir bag) 15 L/min. If airway compromised, intubate.
— Monitor continuously: SaO_2, RR, HR, BP, ECG, temperature.
— Monitor neurology: Pupils – look for fundal haemorrhage/papilloedema, ophthalmoplegia, coma score, posture, tone, reflexes, seizures.
— Shock? Give 20 ml/Kg fluid bolus and reassess (page 47).
— BM <3 mmol/L? Give 2 ml/Kg 10% dextrose (pages 158, 219).
— Seizures (pages 107, 123). Follow guidelines including checking levels of electrolytes (Na^+, Ca^{2+}).
— RICP? Consider mannitol or 3% saline (pages 130, 218).
— Malignant hypertension (page 141)?

— Blood tests: pH, lactate, FBC, U&Es, glucose, Na^+, Ca^{2+}, Mg^{2+}, liver, NH_3, CRP, clotting, ketones, group and save, toxicology, cultures, <u>take 1–2 ml to be frozen and saved</u>.
— Antibiotics: Give cefotaxime, acyclovir, azithromycin: Do not delay if an infection is possible.
— Metabolic? Urgent if: Hypoglycaemia or NH_3 >200 micromol/L or pH < 7.3 + ketones in urine + normal BM. Give 10% dextrose or sodium benzoate (page 157).
— Endocrine and DKA (pages 147, 151)?
— Trauma (pages 161, 165)?
— Urine collection: MCTs, dipstick, ketones, diuresis, toxicology, and take 10ml to be frozen and saved.
— Lumbar puncture: Contraindicated (page 124).
— Urgent CT scan (+/– contrast) once ABCD stabilised. Beware: A normal CT does not exclude RICP.
— Insert an orogastric tube and place on free drainage.
— Commence 2/3 calculated fluid maintenance with 0.9% saline (monitor BM) or 10% dextrose if hypoglycaemic.
— Transport considerations to a PICU: Manage the patient, as per the RICP guidelines (pages 130, 195).

<u>Indications for intubation:</u> **Pages 183–187.**

— Airway compromised or $PaCO_2$ >6KPa or SaO_2 <92% in 15 L/min O_2 or GCS <8 (AVPU <P), obtunded/agitated, shock requiring >40 ml/Kg fluid bolus.
— CT scan: Intubation may be needed for patient safety.
— Status epilepticus unresponsive to early management protocol (page 123).
— Signs of acute RICP (page 130).

COMA SCORES:
GLASGOW COMA SCALE FOR CHILDREN AND AVPU SCALE

GLASGOW COMA SCALE

Best eye response
1. No eye opening
2. Eye opening in pain
3. Eye opening to verbal command
4. Eye opening spontaneously

Best verbal response: Child age/pre-verbal age
1. No vocal response/no response to pain
2. Occasional whimper or moan/mild grimace to pain
3. Cries inappropriately/vigorous grimace to pain
4. Spontaneous irritable cry/response to touch stimuli
5. Alert, communication appropriate for age/normal facial and oro-motor activity

Best motor response
1. No motor response to pain
2. Abnormal extension to pain
3. Abnormal flexion to pain
4. Withdrawal to painful stimuli
5. Localises to painful stimuli or withdraws to touch
6. Obeys command or normal spontaneous movements

AVPU SCALE

Alert
responds to Voice
responds to Pain
Unresponsive

APLS 2012. Resuscitation Council 2010.
**Pediatric Status Epilepticus: treatment and management,
emedicine.medscape.com, 2011.**
Reviewed by Leena Mewasingh, 2014

— Assess ABCD (pages 9–21), temperature, SaO_2, RR, HR, BP, pupils and fontanelle. Call for help? Anaesthetists? PICU?

— Give high flow O_2 15 L/min, face mask with reservoir bag.

— Measure a BM.

— History: **AMPLE** = Allergies, Medications used, Past illnesses, Last meal (evaluate risks of aspiration), Events related to problem.

— Aetiology: **Febrile convulsion? Known epileptic + acute illness? Meningoencephalitis (page 126)? Metabolic (page 155)? Electrolyte abnormalities (glucose, calcium, sodium) (page 107)? Trauma (including NAI) (pages 161, 165, 201)?**

— Duration of fit? Morphology of fit **(generalised, focal)?**

— Treatment given out of hospital? **Midazolam or diazepam*?**

— Blood tests: **Blood gas, electrolytes, FBC, clotting, CRP etc. Toxicology screen? Other tests depend on possible aetiology.**

COMMENTS (see algorithm later)

— * If pre-hospital benzodiazepines have been given, giving more will increase the risks of apnoea. It is therefore recommended that <u>no more than 2 doses be given in total</u>, including the out-of-hospital doses.

— Some patients may have received buccolam: **New pre-filled syringes: 2.5 mg in 0.5 ml, 5 mg in 1 ml, 7.5 mg in 1.5 ml, 10 mg in 2 ml. Buccolam can be <u>given instead</u> of the injection solution of midazolam via the buccal cavity. The pre-filled syringe to choose should be the one containing the dose <u>closest to 0.3 mg/Kg</u> (= dose of the orally given solution of midazolam).**

— Lorazepam supply: **If there is no lorazepam available, midazolam or buccolam should be used.**

— CT Scan? **Intubation may be required to do the CT safely.**

— LP: Rarely contraindicated: **Only contraindicated if there are electrolyte imbalances, signs of RICP, altered consciousness, focal signs, seizure >10 min + GCS <10, clotting disorders, local skin problems.** Measure pressure! **Ask for Gram stain, protein, glucose, PCR, culture and take extra CSF for future tests if they may be needed (page 129).**

— Antibiotics: **(Pages 220, 223) ceftriaxone + consider aciclovir + azithromycin. If ≤1 m: cefotaxime**

+ amoxicillin + consider aciclovir + azithromycin. Always give early even if cause is not immediately clear as infective. Do not wait for an LP.

— Refractory seizures of newborn and infants: **Seek expert advice for possible vitamin B-related encephalopathies or other metabolic disorders. Exclude other causes (page 126). Specific blood and CSF samples will be needed. Pyridoxal 5 phosphate, folinic acid and biotin may be considered.**

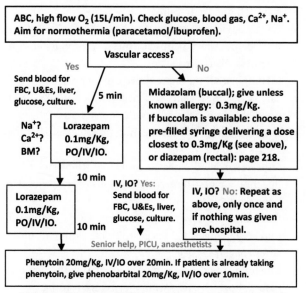

ABC, high flow O_2 (15L/min). Check glucose, blood gas, Ca^{2+}, Na^+. Aim for normothermia (paracetamol/ibuprofen).

Vascular access?

Yes / No

5 min

Send blood for FBC, U&Es, liver, glucose, culture.

Na^+? Ca^{2+}? BM?

Lorazepam 0.1mg/Kg, PO/IV/IO.

Midazolam (buccal); give unless known allergy: 0.3mg/Kg. If buccolam is available: choose a pre-filled syringe delivering a dose closest to 0.3mg/Kg (see above), or diazepam (rectal): page 218.

10 min

Lorazepam 0.1mg/Kg, PO/IV/IO.

10 min

IV, IO? Yes: Send blood for FBC, U&Es, liver, glucose, culture.

IV, IO? No: Repeat as above, only once and if nothing was given pre-hospital.

Senior help, PICU, anaesthetists

Phenytoin 20mg/Kg, IV/IO over 20min. If patient is already taking phenytoin, give phenobarbital 20mg/Kg, IV/IO over 10min.

– Intubation with an anaesthetist (pages 183–187): if thiopental is used, beware of drop in BP. Obtain a PICU bed.
– If signs of RICP: consider RICP protocol (page 130).

MENINGOENCEPHALOPATHY/MENINGITIS/ ENCEPHALITIS

Principles & Practice of Pediatric Infectious Diseases,
3rd ed., Elsevier, 2008.
Reviewed by Hermione Lyall, Alasdair Bamford, 2013

Initial symptoms and clinical signs on examination:
Pages 9–21.

— Can be subtle, non-specific: flu-like illness, vomiting, fatigue, reduced appetite, pyrexial, subpyrexial, headache, lethargy, irritability.

— Can be obviously neurological from the start. Headache, neck pain, reduced consciousness, seizure, focal signs, dizziness, visual loss . . .

— Meningitis: All the signs above can be present.
The typical headache, stiff neck and photophobia are unreliable signs in small children or infants.

— If neurological signs were not present initially, they always develop.

— Other associated signs to look for: Respiratory tract infection or gastrointestinal symptoms, rash, joint or bone pain.

— Deterioration: Low or fluctuating GCS, changes in pupils, signs of RICP (page 130), development of seizures (page 123).

— The following causes can be associated with haemodynamic shock: Sepsis, metabolic, toxins, trauma.

Causes:

In RED are the immediately treatable causes and of dramatic consequence if treatment is slightly delayed. Know the incubation periods for the infections!

— ACUTE INFECTION: *Haemophilus influenzae, E.coli, Meningococcus, Pneumococcus,* Group B Streptococcus, *Staphylococcus, Listeria,* Mycoplasma, *Pertussis, Borrelia* (Lyme disease), *Bartonella, Rickettsia, Shigella, Campylobacter.* Herpes simplex virus, influenza, **enterovirus, adenovirus, parechovirus, measles, mumps, Epstein–Barr virus, HIV,** tuberculosis, leptospirosis, malaria.

— NON-INFECTIOUS: Neurosurgical (tumour, trauma, haemorrhage), sickle cell, poisoning, endocrine, metabolic/electrolyte abnormalities (in particular low glucose, low Ca^{2+}, low Na^+), **hypoxic-ischaemic, NAI (page 201), hyperpyrexic shock, Reye syndrome, inborn errors of metabolism (page 155).**

— VASCULITIS: Systemic lupus erythematosus disease, NMDA receptor antibody encephalitis.

Treatment: **Page 223.**

If suspected, start empirical treatment, before obtaining a diagnosis, for all treatable causes for which delay can have disastrous consequences.

— Ensure stability of ABC: Pages 9–21.
— IV ceftriaxone + IV aciclovir. Add oral azithromycin if there are respiratory symptoms. If <3 m, add

amoxicillin IV (*Listeria*?). Replace ceftriaxone with cefotaxime if patient is requiring Ca^{2+} infusion or if it is a neonate with high bilirubin.

— Consider adding oseltamivir (influenza), anti TB, anti-malarial (page 70), if it seems appropriate.

— Steroids: Give immediately if >3m <u>and</u> if it is likely to be bacterial with an LP showing purulent CSF or WBC > 1000 or raised WBC and protein >1 g/L or bacteria in gram stain.

— IVIG: Not given urgently for meningoencephalopathies. Ensure saved blood samples are taken before giving for future tests that IVIG may alter.

Diagnosis:

CT scan: Urgent for space occupying lesions (bleed, abscess, tumour, hydrocephaly) to identify need for neurosurgery.

History-taking is crucial. In particular, ask the following:

— Immunisations and medications used?

— Travel history: Place, dates, city/countryside, insect bites?

— Contacts: Other sick people, animal contacts, swimming?

— Eating habits? Ingestion of toxins (drugs, plants, medication, pica . . .)?

— Joint/bone pain/rash prior to this episode? When? What?

— Other: Trauma, headaches, family migraine history, haemoglobinopathy, immunosuppression, level of activity, behaviour, confusion?

Blood tests: Gas, glucose, FBC, U&Es, liver test, clotting, albumin, LDH, CK, CRP, ESR, toxicology (page 176), mycoplasma serology + save sample for future tests.

Bacterial cultures: Blood, NPA, throat, urine, stool, CSF.

— CSF: (There are only a few contraindications to LP: page 124) Measure pressure! At least 0.5ml in each tube (except fluoride). Tube 1: Bacterial culture. Tube 2: Save for virology. Tube 3: Protein. Tube 4: Microscopy. (Tube 5: Save for cytospin.) Fluoride tube: Glucose +/− lactate (paired with blood).

— Urine also for pneumococcal antigen, toxicology (page 176).

More specific tests depending on information gathered above.

PCR tests: Choose the most appropriate in discussion with specialist teams (page 223):

— On blood: HSV, enterovirus, paraechovirus, HHV6/7, VZV, EBV, adenovirus, CMV, *Meningococcus*, *Pneumococcus*.

— On CSF: HSV, enterovirus, paraechovirus, HHV6/7, VZV, EBV, adenovirus, CMV, *Meningococcus*, *Pneumococcus*, measles, mumps.

— On NPA: RSV, metapneumovirus, adenovirus, influenza, pertussis.

ACUTELY RAISED INTRACRANIAL PRESSURE (RICP)

Rogers Textbook of Paediatric Intensive Care, 4th ed.,
Williams & Wilkins, 2008.
Dunn, L. *J Neurol Neurosurg Psych*, 2002, 73: i23–i27.
Reviewed by Mehrengise Cooper, 2013

Causes:

Trauma, meningoencephalitis, space occupying lesion (abscess, blood, tumour), hypoxic ischaemic injury. Shock and RICP may be present at the same time complicating management (page 47).

Signs:

Constantly reassess ABCD: Pages 9–21.
— Pale, cold extremities when severe or associated with shock.
— Increased RR → low RR → Cheyne–Stokes breathing (late).
— HR: Initially abnormally high → disproportionately low.
— Prolonged CRT: Present in severe RICP (alone) and or when shock coexists.
— BP: Increased but still within normal range → hypertension when HR drops (high BP, low HR, low GCS: Cushing's syndrome).

— Pulses: Good peripheral pulses (unless shock coexists) and heart sounds normal. Gallop if shock coexists.
— Neuro: GCS, AVPU: abnormal early on (page 121); irritable → lethargic → unconscious. If shock coexists, it is worsened by hypoperfusion due to low BP added to RICP. Abnormal posture/tone? Brisk reflexes? Focal signs? Seizure? Pupils and fontanelle (infant) must be examined regularly throughout: Symmetry? Reaction to light? Size? Fontanelle bulging? Papilloedema (late sign)?
— Blood gas: Respiratory alkalosis → normal → metabolic acidosis if shock coexists. BM low or high depending on stress response.

Comment:

RICP can be associated with haemodynamic shock which renders management difficult because the patient may not be able to keep BP high enough to maintain cerebral blood perfusion. It is important that during the managment, the BP is maintained at normal to high systemic levels (equal or above intracranial pressures) to maintain cerebral blood perfusion. All measures to reduce intracranial pressure must also be used (next page). Intubate early. BP and cardiac function kept stable with careful electrolytic + BM corrections, early inotropes, careful fluid administration (inotropes can be added after 40 ml/Kg of fluids if BP is not stabilised at desired level).

Initial management:

Call senior help, anaesthetists, PICU.

— Oxygen: High flow 15 L/min face mask with reservoir bag.
— Immediate intubation if: AVPU < P or GCS < 8, airway compromised, hypoventilation, obtunded, requires CT, status epilepticus.
   Induction agent for intubation: Ketamine but if patient is in status epilepticus, thiopental is best. Beware of drop in BP with thiopental (page 185).
— Ventilate to $PaCO_2$ 4.5–5.3 KPa.
— Maintain good BP and perfusion: Bolus fluid 10ml/Kg + 10ml/Kg if necessary. Start vasoconstrictors (dopamine peripherally or preferably noradrenaline if central IV access or IO). More fluids may also be needed.
   Stabilise BP above cerebral perfusion pressure: Aim for mean BP above normal systemic (pages 19–23, 47, 217): Mean BP > 65 mm Hg if <2y, mean BP > 70 mm Hg if 2–6y, BP > 80 mm Hg if >6y.
— Keep glucose and electrolytes within normal range (pages 107, 158, 219).
— Aim for ideal Na^+ 145–150 mmol/L.
— Head midline, 30 degrees incline, fluid maintenance restricted to 60% of 0.9% saline.

— Aim for temperature 35–36°C. Avoid hyperthermia. In case of traumatic brain injury, cool within 8 hrs to 32–33°C for 48 hrs and rewarm slowly (page 165).
— Antiacids: Risks of gastric ulcers is higher in brain injury.
— Pain relief/sedation/anaesthesia if needed (page 191).

If signs of worsening RICP:

— Hypertension, bradycardia, abnormal breathing (Cushing's triad) and/or abnormal pupils: Urgent administration of 3% saline or mannitol.
— 3% saline: See page 218 on how to prepare. IV 3 ml/Kg over 5–10 min. Alternatively, use ready-made 2.7% bags if available. Best hyperosmolar effect. Aim for Na^+ level 145–150 mmol/L.
— Mannitol 20% (20g/100ml) may be used: IV 0.25g/Kg over 15min (may be repeated) to 1g/Kg over 30 min. Do not use mannitol in trauma.

Other:

— Antibiotics/antivirals: Ceftriaxone (cefotaxime if <1 m), aciclovir (CNS doses), azithromycin (pages 220, 223).
— Anticonvulsants; phenytoin prophylactically (page 218): Discuss with specialist.
— CT Scan **after** ABCD stabilisation. A normal CT does NOT exclude RICP.

— In case of trauma: **Cervical spine stabilisation (pages 161, 165).**
— NO lumbar puncture **(page 124).**
— Always think of NAI **(pages 201, 206).**

PERSONAL NOTES

RENAL

ACUTE GLOMERULONEPHRITIS (GN)
Reviewed by Jane Deal, 2013

Presence of haematuria (usually visible), proteinuria, raised BP and decreased renal function.

Presentation:

Signs, other than haematuria and proteinuria, may be subtle.
— Oliguria/anuria.
— Hypertension.
— Increasing oedema and ascites.
— Features of the underlying cause.

Causes:

— Post-infectious: Can occur after any acute bacterial or viral infection.
— Vasculitis: Henoch–Schönlein purpura, systemic lupus erythematosus, ANCA-positive vasculitis.
— Post-chronic infections: Infective endocarditis, shunt nephritis, hepatitis B, hepatitis C, HIV.
— Can be associated with other nephropathies: IgA nephropathy, mesangio-capillary GN/membrano-proliferative GN.

Management:

Admission for investigation and monitoring (pages 9–21).

— Investigations: FBC + blood film, ESR, renal profile, liver enzymes, bone profile, C3, C4, ANA, ANCA, anti GBM, immunoglobulins, ASO titre, anti DNAse B.
— Urine: MC&S (+ casts), microalbumin (albumin/creatinine ratio).
— Throat swab for MC&S.
— Fluid balance: Input/output, daily weight.
— Sodium restriction, fluid restriction/diuretics.
— Hypertension: Monitor BP, diuretics, short acting agents (nifedipine).
— Electrolyte disturbances: Restrict potassium and phosphate. Treat as required (page 107).

NEPHROTIC SYNDROME (NS)
Reviewed by Jane Deal, 2013

<u>Definition:</u>

— Heavy proteinuria, hypoalbuminaemia (<25 g/L), oedema, ascites.
— Primary, idiopathic or secondary (e.g. lupus, hepatitis, HIV).
— It can be a relapsing and remitting disease.

<u>Presentation of NS:</u>

— Oedema: Usually short history, dependent, vary in site with posture and time.
— Urine testing: +++ proteinuria.

<u>Complications:</u>

Complications at any stage of NS (i.e. at presentation or during relapses).

— <u>Of the disease:</u> Hypovolaemia, thrombo-embolism, increased susceptibility to infections (pneumococcus, gram negative), severe oedema that can cause organ dysfunction (cellulitis, oliguria…).
— <u>Of treatment:</u> Steroids, other immunosuppressants (cyclophosphamide, ciclosporin A, tacrolimus, mycophenilate mofetil, rituximab).
— <u>Beware of the child with NS who has:</u> Fever, sepsis, peritonitis (page 113), cellulitis, abdominal pain, diarrhoea,

chest pain, headache, drowsiness, vomiting, decreased urine output, worse oedema and ascites. Children with diarrhoea and vomiting and on treatment with tacrolimus/ciclosporin A have a high risk of acute renal failure.

Management of complications:

— Admit + investigations: FBC, haematocrit, renal profile, liver enzymes, amylase. Blood culture. Do a peritoneal tap for MC&S.
— Measure urine sodium: If hypovolaemic, urine sodium is <5 mmol/L.
— Ultrasound of renal tract for evidence of renal vein thrombosis.

Treatment:

— For suspected hypovolaemia: **Ask for advice. 5% HAS (5 g/100ml) 10–20 ml/Kg, IV over 30 min–1h. Do NOT give diuretics.**
— For severe oedema and ascites: **Ask for advice. 20% HAS (20 g/100ml) 2.5–5 ml/Kg, IV over 4–6 h and furosemide (1mg/Kg).**
— If sepsis suspected: **Give IV broad spectrum antibiotics (pages 220, 223).**

MALIGNANT HYPERTENSION
Reviewed by Jane Deal, 2013

Hypertension, papilloedema, vascular haemorrhagic lesions, thickening of small arteries, left ventricular hypertrophy.

Presentation:

— High BP: systolic >99th centile for age, sex, height + 15 mm Hg (pages 9–21).
— Often associated with neurological signs: seizures, drowsiness, decreased GCS, headaches, abnormal vision.

Causes:

Newborn: coarctation, renal artery stenosis, thrombosis.
Older children: Reflux nephropathy, renal artery stenosis, coarctation, haemolytic uraemia syndrome (HUS), glomerulonephritis (GN) (page 137).

Acute management:

— History: Length of symptoms? History of reversible airways disease?
— Examine for causes. Signs of cardiac failure? Neurological status?
— Insert IV line + blood tests: FBC, clotting, renal profile, liver enzymes, calcium, phosphate, alkaline phosphatase, plasma renin and aldosterone. These must be done acutely before any treatment is started.

— Urine M,C&S, catecholamines, microalbumin (albumin/creatinine ratio).
— Chest X-ray, ECG, ultrasound renal tract.
— Monitoring: BP every 15 min + neurological status. Measure urine output and renal function regularly.

Dropping the BP depends on the speed of its rise:

If there is doubt regarding speed of rise of BP, make it drop SLOWLY.

If the rise has been rapid (HUS, acute renal failure, acute GN): BP can be dropped faster.

— Work out target systolic BP based on age/sex/height and BP charts (page 21).
— Subtract target BP from current BP = desired drop in BP. Divide this by 3.
— Aim to drop the BP daily, by a third of the calculated desired drop of BP, for 3 consecutive days.
— If BP falls faster than desired, give IV bolus of 10 ml/Kg 0.9% saline stat.

Drugs: Which to choose (page 220)?

— Labetalol: First choice but contraindications are asthma, cardiac failure.
— Sodium nitroprusside, second best if Labetalol cannot be given.
— Furosemide: 1–2 mg/Kg, IV. Only if there is volume overload in acute renal failure or in GN.
— Nifedipine: Effect is uncertain. Place IV access in case BP drops too fast.

ACUTE RENAL FAILURE
Reviewed by Jane Deal, 2013

Presentation:

— Oliguria/anuria. Beware of polyuric renal failure (renal tract abnormalities).
— Signs of fluid overload.
— Signs of biochemical abnormalities.
— Signs of uraemia.

Causes:

Pre-renal: Cardiovascular failure (hypovolaemia, sepsis, cardiac…), bilateral renal arterial or venous thrombosis, drug toxicity (pages 47, 79–89, 176).

Post-renal: Obstructed solitary kidney, bilateral ureteric obstruction, urethral obstruction, bladder retention.

Renal: Haemolytic uraemia syndrome (HUS), glomerulo-nephritis (page 137).

Tubular: Acute tubular necrosis (ATN), toxins, drugs, hypoxic/ischaemic.

Interstitial causes: Tubular interstitial nephritis, drugs.

Acute on chronic: Decompensation of known chronic renal failure due to intercurrent illness, drugs etc…

Management:

— Blood: FBC, ESR, clotting, renal profile, liver enzymes, bone profile, blood gas, drug levels (e.g. gentamicin).

— Urine: M,C&S, Na$^+$, K$^+$, Cl$^-$, urea, creatinine, microalbumin (if urinalysis is positive for protein).
— Ultrasound of renal tract.

Management to reduce further damage:
— Treat underlying cause.
— May need fluid resuscitation if hypovolaemia is the cause.
— May need frusemide.
— Adapt drug doses to glomerular filtration rate (GFR).

Monitoring: **Measure fluid balance: input/output charting. Consider catheterising the bladder. Daily weight. Continuous BP and cardiac monitor.**

Management:
— Fluid restrict to insensible losses + urine output.
— Treat electrolyte abnormalities: Hyperkalaemia, acidosis (page 107).
— BP management: Pages 141, 220.
— Nutrition: high calories/low potassium intake.
— Renal replacement therapy (dialysis/continuous haemofiltration) if conservative management fails: Development of severe hyperkalaemia, acidosis, uraemia, other biochemical anomalies, volume overload. Renal replacement therapy is also for toxin/drug removal.

PERSONAL NOTES

ENDOCRINOLOGY/METABOLIC

DIABETIC KETOACIDOSIS (DKA)

Rosenbloom A. *Diabetes Therapy*, 2010, 1(2): 103–120.
ISPAD Clinical Practice Concensus Guidelines 2009.
Pediatric Diabetes, 2009, 10 (Suppl 12): 118–133.
Reviewed by Samir Wassouf, Mando Watson, 2012

Discuss all cases with the specialised team.

Diagnosis:

Glycaemia >14 mmol/L + pH <7.30, HCO_3^- <15 mmol/L + ketones. If these are not all present, consider: Hyperosmolar hyperglycaemic non-ketotic syndrome (HHNKS), lactic acidosis, alcoholic ketoacidosis, salicylate overdose, inborn error of metabolism, sepsis.

Definition of HHNKS (rare): BM >33 mmol/L, pH >7.30, HCO_3^- >15 mmol/L, plasma osmolality >320 mOsm/L, small amount ketones, profound dehydration, shock.

Severe DKA: pH < 7.00, HCO_3^- <10 mmol/L, ketones >5 mmol/L, anion gap >16, stupor/coma.

Symptoms: Polyuria, polydipsia, weight loss, various degree of dehydration, rapid RR, Kussmaul breathing, abdominal signs (frequent). Do a BM or dipstix urine for all patients dehydrated with acidosis or with unexplained abdominal signs (pain, vomiting).

History: Is this a new presentation or an acute episode or chronic? What are the usual insulin requirements? Any precipitating cause? Focus of infection?

Degree of dehydration: Page 100. Shock is rare (page 47).

<u>Acute complications:</u>

— Cerebral oedema (+ RICP page 130): Headache, irritability, low HR, <u>rising</u> BP (even if still normal, page 21) or high BP, reduced conscious level.
<u>Risk factors:</u> Presence of a young age, $PaCO_2 < 2KPa$ or high urea at presentation, early start of insulin, too rapid drop of glycaemia and osmolality, administration of HCO_3^-.

— Thrombosis, haemorrhage, infarction: Increased risks in DKA.

<u>Investigations:</u>

Blood tests: Blood glucose, U&E, gas, ketones, FBC, PCV, HbA_1C. For newly diagnosed DKA, add Hb electrophoresis, lactate, islet cell antibodies, anti-GAD antibodies, thyroid function, thyroid antibodies, coeliac antibody screen, vitamin D.
Urine: M, C&S and dipstix. Full septic screen as required.
Calculate osmolality and corrected sodium:

— Serum osmolality (mOsm/L) = $[2 \times (Na^+ + K^+)]$ + blood glucose + urea.

— Corrected Na^+ = Measured Na^+ + $[1.6 \times$ (blood glucose- 5.5)/5.5].

<u>Management:</u>

Monitoring: Weight. Fluid balance/4–6 h. Capillary glucose hrly or more. Hrly blood gas, electrolytes. Capillary or urine ketones/6–12 h. Osmolality + corrected Na^+/6–8h. Continuous SaO_2, ECG, HR. At least hrly RR, BP, CRT, pulses, neurological observations.

Admit to HDU/PICU if: Glucose >50 mmol/L, pH<7.1, severe dehydration + shock, age <2 y, ketones >6 mmol/L, anion gap >16, GCS <12, SaO$_2$ <92%, RICP.

Oxygen 15L/min via face mask with reservoir bag. Only intubate if patient is unable to adequately spontaneously hyperventilate.

NG on free drainage: If the patient is comatose or vomiting.

Fluids:

— If alert and not vomiting: Oral hydration with small frequent volumes.

— If <3% dehydrated: Give maintenance fluid volumes only (page 219).

— If in shock: Give IV 10 ml/Kg 0.9% saline (max 20 ml/Kg). No colloid.

If low BP persists despite 20 ml/Kg 0.9% saline, call PICU.

Avoid IV central line if possible (risks of venous thrombosis).

If IV central access is needed, consider heparinisation.

— When blood volume is restored, calculate fluid requirements over 48 h:

Requirement over 48h = maintenance + deficit – fluid already given.

Deficit (litres) = % dehydration × weight (kg) but do not go above 8%.

Type of fluid and when to change:

— Initially 0.9%NaCl+ 20 mmol KCl in each 500 ml of 0.9%NaCl.

— If glycaemia <14 mmol/L: Change to 5% glucose + 0.45% saline + KCl.

— After 12 h, if Na^+ stable or increasing, use 0.45% saline. If Na^+ low, continue with 0.9% saline. If Na^+ >150 mmol/L slow down the rehydration.

Insulin:

<u>As soon as</u> fluids are started, insulin must start. SC is better and more efficient for mild and moderate DKA.

If SC: 0.2 unit/Kg every 4h, adjusting according to response until basal bolus and carb-counting regimens are started.

If IV: Start at 0.05 unit/Kg/h (page 219) and adjust. Obtain a slow drop of glycaemia (<3–5 mmol/L/h) and of osmolality (<2–3 mOsm/L/h).

If glycaemia <14 mmol/L: change the fluids (as above). Do not reduce insulin rate below 0.03 unit/Kg/h.

If glycaemia rises > 14 mmol/L, increase insulin and do not change the fluids back to normal saline.

If glycaemia <4 mmol/L: 2 ml/Kg 10% dextrose + increase glucose in fluids. Insulin can temporarily be reduced for <u>1h</u>.

If needed, make a solution of 10% glucose + 0.45% saline: 50 ml 50% glucose to 500 ml 0.45% saline/5% glucose.

Electrolytes:

Risks of hypokalaemia. Do not give HCO_3^- (call PICU) (page 109).

ENDOCRINE EMERGENCIES

Donaldson, MD *et al. Archives of Disease in Childhood (Fetal and Neonatal Edition)*, 1994, 70(3): 214–218.

Updated by Michael Coren, 2012

Comments:

— Start treating.
— Seek expert help.
— Diagnostic blood samples <u>must not delay</u> treatment in the presence of severe hypoglycaemia or hypotension.
— When possible, reduce IV steroids to maintenance doses gradually and change to oral administration (see BNF).

Adrenal crisis:

— Rare in children.
— Autoimmune disease, adrenoleukodystrophy, tuberculosis.
— Child on high dose steroids (including inhaled), if these are stopped too rapidly.
— Neonate with ACTH deficiency with hypoglycaemia and jaundice.

Symptoms:

Hypotension, low serum sodium, high potassium.

Management and treatment:

— Take sample for cortisol at presentation.
— Unwell or hypotensive: Give IV 10–20 ml/Kg 0.9% saline (page 47).

— Check BM and treat hypoglycaemia with intravenous glucose (page 219).
— Give hydrocortisone 2 mg/Kg 6 hrly.

Salt-losing newborn with congenital adrenal hyperplasia (CAH):

— Newborns with ambiguous genitalia; common cause of virilisation of girls.
— Salt loss at age 1–4 w after birth, floppy, poor feeding, weight loss.
— Significant hyponatraemia with no obvious cause in a neonate.

Management and treatment:

Treat and do not wait for symptoms nor delay until test results return.

Get blood and urine samples if possible, but never delay treatment.

Sodium deficit is always greater than immediately apparent.

— Unwell or hypotensive: Give IV 10–20 ml/Kg 0.9% saline. Repeat if necessary.
— Check blood glucose. Treat hypoglycaemia with IV glucose (page 219).
— Give 10 mg of hydrocortisone IV 6 hrly.
— Replace sodium with 0.9% saline and change to oral sodium supplements.

Neonatal hypopituitarism:

— Male infants with small genitalia or micropenis.
— Persistent hypoglycaemia.

Steroids must be given even if diagnosis is unclear: these patients can deteriorate rapidly (severe hypoglycaemia). Give 10 mg of hydrocortisone IV 6 hrly.

Steroid cover and steroid dose adjustment for illness and surgery:

The following situations may need steroid dose adjustment for illness and surgery:

— Patients on replacement steroids: adrenal insufficiency, CAH, hypopituitarism.
— Patients on therapeutic steroids: inflammatory bowel disease, post-transplant.
— Anyone who has had high dose steroids in the past 6 months.

If on replacement steroids: If on hydrocortisone the dose should be increased 3 times for 3 days. If on fludrocortisone, no need to change.

If on therapeutic doses of oral steroids: If the patient is able to tolerate oral drugs, there is no need to change the dose.

Adjustments for both groups:

— If the patient is vomiting, not able to take oral therapy or seems to deteriorate, admit the patient and give IV therapy.
— If the patient is unable to tolerate oral therapy and unwell, give hydrocortisone IV 2 mg/Kg, 6 hrly.
— If the patient is well but cannot have oral medication, give a smaller dose.

— If on fludrocortisone, restart the fludrocortisone as soon as oral medication can be tolerated.

Steroid replacement for surgery and anaesthesia:

— Children who require steroid cover should have a dose of intravenous hydrocortisone 2 mg/Kg at induction.
— If patient is unwell and unable to tolerate oral mediation after surgery, give hydrocortisone 2 mg/Kg, 6 hrly.

<u>symptomatic hypoglycaemia:</u>
Possible hyperinsulinism
(pages 158, 219).

METABOLIC EMERGENCIES AND HYPERAMMONAEMIA

British Inherited Metabolic Disease Group,
www.bimdg.org.uk 2008.
Auron, A, Brophy, PD. *Pediatr Nephrol*,
2012, 27: 207–222.
CATS (Children Acute Transport Service), 2013.
Summary by Claudine De Munter and Michael Carter

Presentation:

Encephalopathy, seizures and apnoea, unexplained metabolic acidosis, hypoglycaemia, cardiac failure/cardiomyopathy, liver dysfunction.

Initial management:

Contact a specialist in metabolic medicine when suspected. A transfer to a specialist centre may be necessary.
Monitor continuously SaO_2, RR, HR, BP, neurology at least hrly initially.

— Treat seizures and reduced consciousness: Pages 119–123.
— Give a fluid bolus: 10 ml/Kg saline 0.9%.
  If in shock, repeat bolus ± inotropes (pages 47, 217).
— Promote an anabolic state: Stop protein intake for maximum 36–48 h (reduce production of toxins). Give hypercaloric glucose infusions: IV 10% dextrose ± electrolytes; at least 5 mg/Kg/min (=3 ml/Kg/h).

If dehydrated: Calculate maintenance + deficit (pages 99, 101). Give 1/3 over 6 h and the rest over 24 h.

May need dextrose >10% (12.5%, 20%) to give through a central IV line.

— Hypoglycaemia <3 mmol/L: Give immediate oral or IV 2 ml/Kg dextrose 10% then an infusion to maintain euglycaemia (see below).

Monitor BM hrly. May need dextrose >10% (12.5% or 20%) to give through a central IV line.

— Investigations: Blood samples for a gas (including pH, glucose, lactate), ammonia, plasma ketones, clotting, plasma amino acids, blood spot acyl carnitine profile, U&Es, FBC, CRP, liver function, blood culture.

— Urine tests: Dipstix, ketones, organic acids, culture.

— If hyperglycaemia: Give insulin (see DKA, page 147). Do not reduce glucose intake.

— Metabolic acidosis: Give fluids or HCO_3^- (pages 47, 109). Monitor blood Na^+.

— Hyperammonaemia: See further for management (page 157).

— Treat any sign of infection aggressively to avoid rapid catabolic decompensation.

<u>Indications for intubation:</u> **Pages 183–187.**

Low conscious level, intractable seizures, apnoea, shock.

HYPERAMMONAEMIA

Normal: NH_3 <50 micromol/L.

Management: **as above.**

— Urgent treatment: If NH_3>150 micromol/L in neonates, or NH_3 >100 micromol/L in infant.

— If NH_3 >200 micromol/L: Give an infusion of sodium benzoate + phenylbutyrate: 250 mg/Kg of each over 90 min then 20 mg/Kg/h.

  Preparation of a sodium benzoate + phenylbutyrate infusion: Dilute 250 mg/Kg of each drug in 15 ml/Kg of 5% or 10% dextrose. The concentration must be <2 g/50 ml. Monitor Na^+ level: 1 g sodium benzoate and 1 g phenylbutyrate contain 7 mmol and 5.4 mmol Na^+ respectively.

— Haemofiltration: Contact a PICU or a nephrologist if: NH_3 >200 micromol/L after 6 h of treatment or if NH_3 level >300 micromol/L.

— Treat any infection.

Causes:

— Congenital: If there is no associated acidosis: urea cycle enzyme defects. If acidosis is associated: Organic acidurias, fatty acid oxidation defects, congenital lactic acidosis.

— Acquired: Transient hyperammonaemia of the newborn, Reye syndrome, liver failure, valproate therapy, severe systemic illness.

SYMPTOMATIC HYPOGLYCAEMIA

Do not delay treatment. Monitor BM during treatment and until stable.

Investigations:

If there are samples of blood at presentation: measure lactate, insulin, cortisol, growth hormone, free fatty acids, fluoride oxalate, ketones, acyl-carnitine profile, amino and organic acids in plasma.

Obtain the first urine: dipsticks, ketones, amino acids, organic acids.

Treatment:

Give 2 ml/Kg of 10% dextrose slow IV bolus, followed by an infusion of 10% dextrose. More concentrated glucose solutions need a central IV line. Check BM hrly with a ward-based monitor and aim for a glucose level within the normal range.

...with suspected hyperinsulinism:

Give continuous oral feeds rather than bolus feeds.

If maximum oral intake is given and the child remains hypoglycaemic, continue with a combination of oral and IV fluids. Increase the glucose input to 12.5% or 15% glucose which must be given via an IV central line.

Glucagon or octreotide are further therapeutic options.

PERSONAL NOTES

INJURY

PAEDIATRIC TRAUMA
ATLS 2010, APLS 2012,
ATLS 2008, APLS 2010.
Sabeena Qureshi, Rebecca Salter, 2012

— Blunt trauma: most common mechanism of injury in children.

— Traumatic brain injury is most common serious traumatic injury.

— A child's skeleton being incompletely calcified, internal organ damage is often noted without bone fractures.

— Up to 30% reduction of circulating blood volume may be required to decrease the systolic blood pressure.

— <u>All children</u> including small infants and children with Down's syndrome are at high risk of cervical spine injuries.

<u>The trauma team leader (TTL) is always in charge.</u>
Before the patient arrives:

— Introduce yourself to the TTL: Name, speciality, grade and sign in.

— Ascertain type of trauma coming in and stability of patient.

— If the major haemorrhage protocol is activated (page 173) or patient is unstable or likely to be bleeding, inform a consultant and PICU.

— Estimate the weight of the patient (page 246), calculate drug doses, ETT sizes (page 184).
— Write this information on the white board.
— Put on gloves, lead apron (+/− plastic apron), +/− goggles.
— Keep noise to a minimum. Direct questions or information to the TTL.

What happens at a trauma call
(order interchangeable):

— Patient arrives and everyone listens to the handover.
— Scoop out/off spinal board or vacumat.
— Continue full spinal precautions (collar, in-line stabilisation).
— Monitoring on.
— Primary survey.
— IV access, bloods, venous gas, thromboelastograph (TEG) if applicable.
— Apply splints.
— FAST scan (focussed assessment sonography for trauma).
— X-rays (chest, pelvis, C-spine).
— Log roll and complete examination (including the back).
— Further imaging (CT scans, angiography, plain films...).
— Secondary survey.
— Life-saving interventions at any stage.
— Stand down when instructed by TTL. Write notes +/− drug chart.

<u>Role of the paediatrician at the trauma call:</u>

This will be designated by the TTL. It may include the following:

— Primary survey.
— Talk to patient/relative, reassure, ascertain if there is any pain, history of event, past medical history, drug history, allergies, last meal, anaesthetic history.
— Assist with IV access, bloods, venous gas and TEG sample if requested. Label the bloods properly (including a handwritten X-match sample) and send them off.
— Do not give any fluids unless instructed to do so by the TTL. Colloid should not be used.
— Scribe: It is best to have familiarised oneself in advance with the trauma documentation.
— Thoracostomies and chest drain insertion for pneumothorax +/− haemothorax which may be present in the absence of rib fractures.
— Accompany to CT scan and back.
— If the paediatrician is stood down by the TTL, all documentation must be completed in the trauma notes, including the times on the signing-in sheet.
— Complete the clerking and drug chart if the child is to be admitted under the paediatric team.

If an adolescent (<16 y) is admitted to the Major Trauma Ward: The paediatric team, including the consultant, must review the patient at least daily and document in the notes (with bleep numbers). Any child admitted to any of the wards must be under a named paediatric consultant.

Consider safeguarding issues: **Make appropriate referrals to social care/police. These need to be followed up with a written CAF form, available in A&E. If there are safety issues but no safeguarding concerns, a health visitor referral form must be completed for the liaison health visitor in paediatric A&E (pages 201, 206, 210).**

PAEDIATRIC TRAUMATIC BRAIN INJURY
CATS (Children Acute Transport Service) 2011.
ATLS 2010, APLS 2012.
Traumatic brain injury, *Pediatric Critical Care Medicine*, 2012: http://journals.lww.com/pccmjournal/ toc/2012/01001
Summary by Claudine De Munter

Refer to page 161.
<u>Assessment:</u> **Pages 9–21.**

— Time and mechanism of injury.
— Loss of consciousness at scene and subsequently.
— Resuscitation at scene and subsequently.

Clinical signs to look out for:

— GCS variations, airway reflexes, pupillary response.
— Signs of basal skull fracture: haemotympanium, 'panda' eyes (periorbital ecchymosis), CSF otorrhoea, Battle's sign (ecchymosis of the mastoid process).
— External signs including skull fractures.
— Post-traumatic seizures.
— Vomiting.
— Amnesia.
— Assessment of spinal cord function: movement of limbs, priapism, spinal shock.

In particular, while maintaining <u>full spinal precautions</u>:

— Monitor for SaO_2, RR, HR, BP continuously.

— Do blood gases, routine blood tests (include clotting, X-match).
— Secondary survey to do with senior orthopaedic and general surgeons.
— Trauma imaging: Do an abdominal assessment with a FAST scan +/– CT.
— Do not forget the possibility of NAI (pages 201–206).

Criteria for referral to ICU and neurosurgery include:

— GCS < 8 after initial resuscitation.
— Unexplained confusion for more than 4 h.
— Deteriorating GCS.
— Progressive focal neurological signs.
— Seizure without full recovery.
— Suspected penetrating injury; CSF leak.

Initial management:

Stabilisation of airway and cervical spine, breathing and circulation are priorities <u>before attention to other injuries</u>.

— Suspicion of cervical spine injury: GCS < 15 at any time, neck pain or tenderness, focal neurological deficit, paraesthesia.
— If cardiovascularly unstable, requiring volume resuscitation: Consider other sites of blood loss: chest, abdomen, pelvis, limbs (page 173).
— At least 2 good venous lines: X-match blood.
— Transfuse to Hb > 10 g/dL.
— Pass urinary catheter and <u>orogastric</u> tube.
— Perform secondary survey.

— Consider NAI (pages 201–206).
— <u>Indications for CT scanning:</u> GCS ≤ 13 at any time since injury, GCS ≤ 14 at 2 h after injury, suspected open or basal skull fracture, post-traumatic seizure, focal neurological deficit, more than 1 episode vomiting, amnesia of events that occured more than 30 min before the impact, presence of coagulopathy.
— <u>Cervical spine imaging:</u>
  Plain films; C7-T1 junction (may require Swimmer's view).
  Do a CT of the neck if intubated to obtain better and adequate high spine views.
— <u>Antibiotics:</u> If there is a CSF leak or a penetrating head injury: Give co-amoxiclav 30 mg/Kg or cefuroxime 30 mg/Kg + metronidazole 7.5 mg/Kg.

<u>Indications for intubation:</u> **Pages 183–187.**

— GCS < 8.
— Loss of airway reflexes.
— Ventilatory insufficiency: PaO_2 < 9 KPa in air or PaO_2 < 13 KPa in oxygen or $PaCO_2$ > 6 KPa.
— Spontaneous hyperventilation ($PaCO_2$ < 3.5 KPa): Possible RICP? (Page 130.)
— Significant maxillofacial injury.
— Copious bleeding into mouth.
— Seizures.

<u>Post-intubation:</u> **Pages 130, 187.**

— Maintain in-line immobilisation of cervical spine, head at 30°.

— Well oxygenated and ventilated to $PaCO_2$ 4.5–5.3 KPa.
— High normal mean BP (noradrenaline): Mean BP> 65 mm Hg if <2y, mean BP>70 mm Hg if 2–6y, mean BP>80 mm Hg if >6y.
— Glucose in normal range.
— Phenytoin prophylactically.
— 3% saline (or ready-made 2.7% saline) if there are signs of RICP.
— Temperature: Cool within 8 hrs to 32–33 °C for 48 hrs, rewarm slowly.
— Ranitidine or Omeprazole: For high risk of stress ulcers.

CHILDREN'S BURNS GUIDELINES
London and South East England Burn Network (LSEBN), 2010:
www.lsebn.nhs.uk/downloads/

Referral criteria for Specialised Burns Units:

— All >30% total body surface area (TBSA) with partial thickness (PT).
— All >20% TBSA with full thickness (FT).
— All >15% TBSA and <1 y old.
— All FT circumferential burns.
— All burns on face, hands, feet, perineum.
— All neonatal burns.
— If >10%: discuss with a specialised Burn's Unit.
— Burns with no other injury: **Refer to a Burn's Unit.**
— Burns + endotracheal intubation: **Refer to a Burn's** Unit with Intensive Care support.
— Burns + other injuries (**ex. trauma**): Discuss choice for the best PICU.
— Inhalation injury, minor surface burn, no head injury: Patient can be admitted to a general PICU.

Mechanism and time: **Time? Hot fluid? Caustic? Electrical? Explosive? Flame? Smoke inhalation? Consider NAI (pages 201–206).**

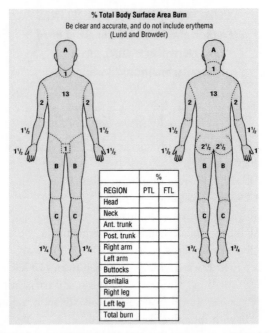

% Total Body Surface Area Burn
Be clear and accurate, and do not include erythema
(Lund and Browder)

REGION	% PTL	FTL
Head		
Neck		
Ant. trunk		
Post. trunk		
Right arm		
Left arm		
Buttocks		
Genitalia		
Right leg		
Left leg		
Total burn		

Area	Age 0	1	5	10	15	Adult
A = ½ OF HEAD	9½	8½	6½	5½	4½	3½
B = ½ OF ONE THIGH	2¾	3¼	4	4½	4½	4¾
C = ½ OF ONE LOWER LEG	2½	2½	2¾	3	3¼	3½

Management:

— High flow oxygen: 15 L/min face mask with reservoir bag.
— Call anaesthetists if there is stridor and if there are facial burns <u>before swelling develops</u>.
— Full secondary survey, look for other lesions (page 161).

— Monitor SaO$_2$, RR, HR, BP, CRT, pulses, blood gas (pages 9–21).
— Do BM, routine blood tests including FBC, X-match.
— ECG for electric burns.
— Cyanide levels (if there is a metabolic acidosis or if in coma): Treat if level >3 mg/L.
— Cervical spine immobilisation if trauma.
— Prophylactic antibiotics not recommended.
— Cover burns with cling film.
— Pain management: Obtain anaesthetic advice (page 191).
— Urinary catheter: All >20% TBSA and <u>all</u> perineal burns. Aim for an output >2 ml/Kg/h if there is a risk of rhabdomyolysis (electrical burns or trauma).

Fluids:

— If >10% TBSA: Obtain good IV access.
— If >30% TBSA: Place at least 2 IV cannulae.
— Resuscitation fluids (RF): **All >10% TBSA: Use the Parkland formula with Hartmann's solution: 4 ml × weight in Kg × %burn over 24 hrs with 1/2 over the first 8 hrs and 1/2 over the next 16 hrs.**
— Maintenance IV or feeding, <u>in addition to</u> resuscitation fluids (RF):

• All <3 months with <20% TBSA: Feed as normal in addition to RF.
• All <3 months with ≥20% TBSA: Add maintenance fluids in addition to RF. Use 0.45% NaCl + 5% glucose. GIve a volume equal to daily requirements.
• All >3 months: Nil by mouth. No need to add any more fluid to the RF.

<u>Intubation:</u> **Pages 32, 183, 187.**

— Airway burns and smoke inhalation: ALL require prophylactic endotracheal intubation even if breathing is normal initially. Airway swelling may develop rapidly.
— All with $FiO_2 > 0.5$, electric shock, severe metabolic acidosis, burns with major trauma, severe shock, GCS < 8 or fluctuating.
— Give 100% oxygen until CO < 10%.*
— Ventilation pressures required can be high if pneumonitis or ARDS develop or if the chest wall becomes rigid due to the burns.

*Carboxy Hb levels (blood gas):

<8% normal in smokers.
>15% severe exposure.
>20% hyperbaric oxygen.

PAEDIATRIC MAJOR HAEMORRHAGE CLINICAL PATHWAYS (<50 Kg)

Sabeena Qureshi, 2012

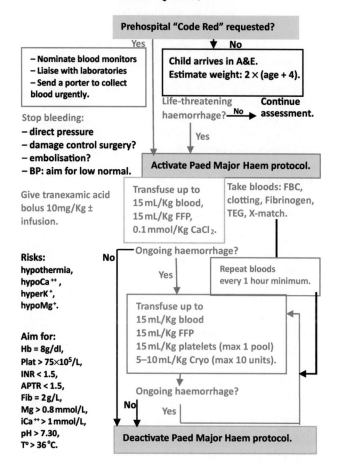

Prehospital "Code Red" requested?

Yes — No

- Nominate blood monitors
- Liaise with laboratories
- Send a porter to collect blood urgently.

Child arrives in A&E.
Estimate weight: 2 × (age + 4).

Stop bleeding:

- direct pressure
- damage control surgery?
- embolisation?
- BP: aim for low normal.

Life-threatening haemorrhage? — No → **Continue assessment.**

Yes

Activate Paed Major Haem protocol.

Give tranexamic acid bolus 10mg/Kg ± infusion.

Transfuse up to 15 mL/Kg blood, 15 mL/Kg FFP, 0.1 mmol/Kg $CaCl_2$.

Take bloods: FBC, clotting, Fibrinogen, TEG, X-match.

Risks: hypothermia, $hypoCa^{++}$, $hyperK^+$, $hypoMg^+$.

No — Ongoing haemorrhage?

Yes

Repeat bloods every 1 hour minimum.

Aim for:
Hb = 8g/dl,
Plat > 75×10⁵/L,
INR < 1.5,
APTR < 1.5,
Fib = 2g/L,
Mg > 0.8mmol/L,
iCa^{++} > 1mmol/L,
pH > 7.30,
T° > 36°C.

Transfuse up to
15 mL/Kg blood
15 mL/Kg FFP
15 mL/Kg platelets (max 1 pool)
5–10 mL/Kg Cryo (max 10 units).

Ongoing haemorrhage?

No — Yes

Deactivate Paed Major Haem protocol.

PAEDIATRIC MAJOR HAEMORRHAGE PROTOCOL (<50 Kg)
Imperial College Healthcare NHS Trust Haematology Team

— Rapid blood loss with shock or with no likelihood of control.
— Anticipated or actual administration of 40 mL//Kg of blood.

Refer to the local major haemorrhage protocol. The following is based on the Imperial College Healthcare NHS Trust's protocol.
Call Emergency number. Say 'Major Paediatric Haemorrhage'.
Say hospital name and area. Call the Blood Transfusion Laboratory:

<u>Information needed by the Blood Transfusion Laboratory:</u>

— Paediatric major haemorrhage protocol being activated.
— Patient identification: Hospital/A&E number, name and date of birth.
— Patient location. Approximate weight.
— Name and contact details of person activating protocol.
— Cause of bleeding.
— How urgently (in minutes) until blood is needed at the bedside.
— Group and save, FBC and coagulation screen samples being sent. If difficulty obtaining blood samples, ensure a 4 mL EDTA sample is sent for X-match as a priority.

— Emergency O negative blood in units if required.
— OR group-specific blood (*O negative if blood group unknown*) according to the volume in ml/Kg required.
— OR X-matched blood, *if there is a currently valid sample available* and according to the volume in ml/Kg required.
— FFP (after 30 minutes of thawing) according to the volume in ml/Kg required.

Aiming to administer volumes as BLOOD 1.5: FFP 1.

Once these components are collected from the laboratory:

Further blood and FFP will be automatically prepared according to the volume in ml/Kg required.

At this stage consider:

— Platelets 15ml/Kg (up to 1 pack).
— Cryoprecipitate 5 – 10ml/Kg (up to 10 single-donor units).

The lab will continue to issue volumes of blood and FFP while the patient is bleeding.

Ensure a porter is sent to collect blood and components.

Availability of blood for collection:

— Emergency O negative blood: Immediate.
— Group-specific blood: 10 minutes.
— X-matched blood: 45 minutes.
— Fresh frozen plasma: 30 minutes to thaw.
— Cryoprecipitate: 15 minutes to thaw.
— Platelets: Immediate if on site but replacement delivery up to 2 hours.

POISONING
APLS 2012.
Updated by David Inwald, Rebecca Salter, 2013

National Poisons Centre or Toxbase (www.toxbase.org)

History:

— Name, dosage, amount ingested, time and date of ingestion.
— Route of poisoning (oral or injection), geographic location.
— Intentional or unintentional and details (pages 201–206).
— Suicide attempt: Even if trivial, admit for psychiatric assessment (page 205).
— Past history: Other episodes, medical history, medications, psychiatric history.
— Terrorism: Consider poisoning with chemical or biological agents.

Emergency assessment and stabilisation:

— Remove contaminated clothing and assess ABC (pages 9–21) + SaO_2.
— High flow O_2 (15 L/min, mask with reservoir bag), ensure airway patency.

— Beware of changes of consciousness that will increase the risk of aspiration. Intubate if there is a poor gag reflex, GCS ≤8 or fluctuating (page 119).

— BP, HR at least hrly until monitoring is no longer necessary.

— ECG: If poisoning is unclear and for all cardiotoxic drugs (tricyclics…).

— Dysrhythmias and DC shock may be needed (pages 28, 218).

— Conscious child should be anaesthetised first.

— DC shock may be dangerous in digoxin poisoning.

— Antiarrhythmics may be used on advice from a poisons centre.

— Shock: Fluid boluses ± inotropes (beware, they are proarryhthmic) (pages 47, 216, 217).

— Conscious level: Monitor hrly with other neurological observations.

— Treat convulsions with a benzodiazepine (pages 123, 218).

— Check BM. Hypoglycaemia? Give 2–5 ml/Kg, 10% dextrose (pages 158, 219).

— Give Naloxone (Narcan®) if altered mental status: IV, IM, in ETT; 0.01 mg/Kg, repeated if needed, max 2 mg. Then infusion of 0.01 mg/Kg/h.

Further investigations:

— **Anion gap >16:** Methanol, ethanol, alcohol, salicylates, ketones, iron.

— **Osmolar gap >20:** Methanol, ethylene glycol (page 246).

— **Blood tests:** FBC, U&E, liver and renal function.
— **Blood levels:** Acetaminophen, salicylates, ethanol, ethylene glycol, isopropyl alcohol, digoxin, iron, lithium, theophylline, anticonvulsants and methanol.
— **Urine for toxicology:** 'Sure Step' urine drug cards: amphetamines, barbiturates, benzodiazepines, ecstasy, methadone, morphine, tricyclics, cannibis.
— **Chest X-ray:** If aspiration, coma, non-cardiogenic pulmonary oedema due to salicylates, narcotics, paraquat, sedative-hypnotics.
— **Abdominal X-ray** for drug packets, salicylates, calcium, iron, radiopaque objects. Hydrocarbons give an image of a 'layer' between gastric fluid and gastric air bubble.

Determination of ingested substance(s):

— **Stimulants:** Mydriasis, tremor, tachycardia, irritable, diaphoresis, mania, fits, arrhythmias:
Cocaine, amphetamines, caffeine, theophylline, tricyclic antidepressants, antihistamines and hallucinogens.
— **Depressants:** Lethargy, low GCS, myosis, hypothermia, coma:
Alcohol, benzodiazepines, barbiturates, muscle relaxants, chloral hydrate.
— **Pupils constricted:** Opioids (heroin, morphine), cholinesterase inhibitors (organophosphate insecticides, carbamate insecticides).

— **Pupils dilated:** Anticholinergic drugs (atropine, benztropine), antihistamines, orphenadrine, thioridazine, tricyclic antidepressants.
— **Dilated pupils and blindness:** Quinine and methanol.

Decontamination procedures:

Syrup of ipecac should NOT be used.

Gastric lavage: Mostly beneficial within 1 h of ingestion.

— Patient must be able to protect the airway (+ good gag reflex) or else intubate with ETT.
— Contraindications: Alkalis (sodium hydroxide), acids (sulphuric, hydrochloric), hydrocarbons, patient not fully alert, airway not protected, or no gag reflexes and not intubated.
— Complications: Aspiration, perforation of the oesophagus or bronchus.
— Method: NG tube (28 – 36 Fr); 0.9% saline in 15ml/Kg aliquots until clear.

Activated charcoal:

— Not useful for alcohol, iron, fluorides, potassium, lithium, methanol, ethylene glycol.
— Repeat doses for aspirin, barbiturates and theophylline.
— It can be drunk or given via NG or a lavage tube after gastric washout.

— Risks: Lung damage if aspirated. <u>Airway protection</u> is important.
— Dose: Usually 500 mg – 1 g/Kg, once or up to 4 hrly + osmotic laxative with the first dose. Give smaller amounts hrly if vomiting.
— Consider antiemetic (cyclizine 0.5 – 1 mg/Kg IV or ondansetron 0.1 mg/Kg by slow IV).

PERSONAL NOTES

ANAESTHETICS/PAIN/TRANSPORT OF PATIENTS

HELPING THE ANAESTHETIST
TO GET READY TO INTUBATE
APLS 2012.
Updated by David Inwald, Sabeena Qureshi, 2012

— Trained staff only.
— Preparation, equipment, monitoring are essential.
— Preoxygenate: Mask with reservoir bag (15L/min O_2) and tight-fitting face mask sized to child's face for bag/mask ventilation.
— Bag: Self-inflating Ambu bag and if possible a Jackson Rees circuit (Ayre's T-piece).
— Stethoscope.
— Guedel oral airways: Sized from corner of mouth to angle of jaw.
— Suction: Yankauer, suction catheters. Put suction on maximum.
— Monitoring: ECG, SaO_2, BP (every 2 minutes), oxygen analyser for inspired oxygen (FiO_2), end-tidal CO_2 (capnography to confirm ETT placement and assess cardiac output).
— Intravenous access: 1 or 2 confirmed working IV cannulae.
— AMPLE: Allergies? Medications used? Past illnesses? Last meal? Last drink? Solids? Events related to problem? Anaesthetic history?
— Blood gas: pH, PCO_2, PO_2, BD, HCO_3^-, Na^+, K^+, Ca^{++}, lactate, Hb.

— NG tube? May be needed before induction. Discuss with anaesthetist. If bagging with a face mask/Ambu bag, place NG tube on free drainage and aspirate air regularly with a syringe (reduce risks of aspiration).

— Emergency drugs for cardiovascular complications of induction: Mainly bradycardia or cardiac arrest.

— Fluid bolus 10–20 ml/Kg 0.9% saline: Pre-load if possible to help reduce risks of dropping BP/cardiac arrest on induction.

— Two laryngoscope blades: Robert-Shaw/Seward/Miller: Straight blade preferred in neonates/infants. Macintosh: Curved blade for the older child.

— Endotracheal tubes (ETT): Choose 3 sizes: Ideal size + one ETT 0.5 size over + one ETT 0.5 size under. Choosing ideal size (internal diameter in mm): >1y: age/4 + 4 if <u>un</u>cuffed and age/4 + 3.5 if cuffed; infants: 3.5–4; neonates: 3.0–3.5; premature infants: 2–3.5. Use lubricating gel for all.
Length of ETT: Oral ETT, at lips: <1y: 3x ETT size (cm); >1y: 12 + Age/2. Nasal ETT, at nostril: >1y: 15 + age/2.

— Bougie and stylet + Magill forceps to guide nasal ETT/NG tube or remove objects.

— Laryngeal masks: To use for difficult bag/mask ventilation or intubation.

— Tube tie/tape: Cut tapes: Melbourne strapping. ▰▰▰◣

— Prepare induction drugs: See below.

— Direct laryngoscopy: Pre-oxygenation. Check that it is possible to oxygenate and ventilate with bag/mask ventilation *before* giving induction and paralysing drugs. Focus on oxygenation rather than intubation.

Give induction and paralysis. When the child is anaesthetised (+/–1min), use the laryngoscope blade gently, pull along axis to see the glottis. Do not rotate. The risks are injuries to gums and teeth, mucosal swelling and bleeding. Beware of risks of aspiration of stomach content. <u>Straight blade</u>: Place in upper oesophagus. <u>Curved blade</u>: Place tip in the vallecula, above the epiglottis. Feed the lubricated ETT into the right side of the mouth. Turning it so the curve is initially horizontal prevents it obscuring the view. Ask assistant for cricoid pressure to help visualise the larynx. Record the ease and the view obtained.

— Check tube placement, ventilation and oxygenation: Mist in ETT, chest rise, end-tidal CO_2, SaO_2, auscultation, chest X-ray, blood gas.

Problems that may occur:

— If you have failed 3 attempts at intubation, stop! Focus on <u>oxygenation</u> via bag/mask ventilation. Call for senior help.
— Dropping/rising BP, HR: Treat as required.
— Aspiration of gastric content: The risk is reduced with gentle bag/mask ventilation, NG tube, or gentle cricoid pressure with anaesthetic advice.

Drugs:

Often rapid sequence intubation (RSI) drugs are needed. Sometimes (e.g. upper airways obstruction) gas inhalation is the preferred method of induction (in theatres).

— Induction IV: The contraindications and side effects need to be known.

Thiopental 2 mg/Kg: Anti-fitting action. Risk drop in BP and cardiac output.

Ketamine 2 mg/Kg: Good as bronchodilator and for haemodynamic instability. <u>Not</u> contraindicated in head trauma or RICP.

— Paralysis IV: The contraindications and side effects need to be known.

<u>Short acting:</u> Suxamethonium 1–2 mg/Kg, rapid. Never use in any musculoskeletal disorder (risks of hyperkalaemia).

<u>Long acting:</u> Vecuronium 0.1 mg/Kg. Reversed by neostigmine: 50 microgr/Kg, max 2.5 mg.

Other: Atracurium 0.5 mg/Kg, rocuronium 1 mg/Kg.

— Maintenance IV: Fentanyl 1 microgr/Kg; morphine 0.1mg/Kg; midazolam 0.1 mg/Kg.

HELPING THE ANAESTHETIST
VENTILATE AND OXYGENATE
Rogers Textbook of Paediatric Intensive Care,
4th ed., Williams & Wilkins, 2008.
Claudine De Munter, Ruchi Sinha, 2012

<u>General Management following intubation:</u> **Page 183.**

Continuous monitoring: SaO_2, RR, HR, BP, End-tidal CO_2, blood gases.

Choose pressure limited ventilation.

The following is a guide of what can be done if there are no particular requirements:

— Start with PIP 20–23 cm H_2O. Modify PIP according to end-tidal CO_2, SaO_2, blood gases/20–30 min and aim for a tidal volume of 5–7ml/Kg.
— Choose a rate that is physiological for age.
— Choose an I:E ratio of 1:2 (unless patient is asthmatic, see below).
— Choose an inspiratory time: 0.8–1.0 sec for children, 0.6–0.75 sec for babies.
— Start with PEEP 5 cm H_2O.
— Start with $FiO_2 = 1$. Reduce it if SaO_2 is stable above 93%.
— Use end-tidal CO_2 to monitor ventilation. Correlate it with an arterial $PaCO_2$ (blood gas). Allow $PaCO_2$ to rise as long as $7.25 \leq pH \leq 7.5$.
— Sedate: Morphine and midazolam infusions ± paralysis.
— If BP is high: Lack of sedation? Pain (HR high too?) Neurological (HR high or low)? Hypervolaemia (HR not high)?

— If BP is low: Hypovolaemia (HR high)? Excess of sedation (causing vasodilatation)? Cardiac cause (HR high or low)? Electrolyte/metabolic imbalance (HR varies)? Sepsis (HR high too)? Tamponnade (pneumothorax)?

Asthma: Page 38.

— Intubate with a cuffed ETT (if high ventilation pressures are required).
— Induction and paralysis: Ketamine 2 mg/Kg (bronchodilatation), OR inhalational agents (bronchodilatation) and suxamethonium 2 mg/Kg. Contraindications and side effects must be known (page 185).
— Fentanyl/midazolam/ketamine/vecuronium: To sedate and paralyse.
— Avoid morphine or atracurium (histamine release).
— Give fluid boluses for dropping BP on induction (10–20 ml/Kg).

Management following intubation:

— Allow for permissive hypercapnia (let CO_2 rise as long as pH >7.25).
— Rate: Choose a slower than physiological rate with a long expiration (I:E 1:2, 1:3).
— Use a PEEP 5–7 cm H_2O to counteract the intrinsic PEEP and avoid air trapping.
— Physiotherapy for mucous plugging. Salbutamol nebulisers.
— Risks if high airway pressure: Pneumothorax and compromised venous return. Both lead to hypotension.

Give fluid bolus. A chest drain if air leaks develop may need to be placed.

Anaphylaxis: **Page 50.**

— If there is airway obstruction: Call urgent senior anaesthetic and ENT.
— Intubation in theatres and an inhalational induction will be used.
— Patient may require a tracheostomy.
— Ventilation: Similar to asthma protocol.
— If there is a persistent hypotension/bronchospasm: Start an adrenaline infusion (as per protocol).
— Give NaHCO$_3$ 1mmol/Kg over 1 hour, if the base deficit >10 and pH<7.2, despite appropriate treatment.

Shock: **Page 47.**

Summary:

— Choose a rapid sequence with ketamine (maintains BP).
— Risks of losing cardiac output during induction are higher with inhalation agents, thiopental, propofol and increase if hypovolaemia is severe, and if there is low K$^+$, low Ca^{2+}, severe metabolic acidosis (pH <7.2).
— Once intubated: FiO$_2$ 1 with PEEP ≥5 cm H$_2$O (max 10 cm H$_2$O) to control pulmonary oedema (capillary leak) and improve recruitment particularly if more fluid boluses are needed for the BP. Inotropes and metabolic corrections (clotting, electrolytes, glucose, bicarbonate) will also be ongoing.

Duct-dependent cardiac lesion: **Page 83.**

When intubated, keep FiO_2 to the level necessary to maintain SaO_2 75–80% (use FiO_2 between 0.21 and 1).

Neurological:
Coma, RICP, status epilepticus, head trauma:
Pages 119–123, 130, 165.

Summary:

— Head trauma: Maintain in-line immobilisation of cervical spine.
— Induction: Ketamine or thiopental (an anti-convulsant but risks dropping BP).
— Sedation: Midazolam infusion (anti-convulsant).
— If there are signs of RICP: Obtain SaO_2>95%. Ventilate to $PaCO_2$ (4.5–5.3KPa). Maintain mean BP to high normal levels. Use fluids bolus and early use of noradrenaline. Keep mean BP >55 mm Hg if <2y, >60 mm Hg if 2–6y, >70 mm Hg if >6y.
— Keep glucose in normal range.
— Use phenytoin prophylactically.
— Use mannitol or 3% saline (or ready-made 2.7% saline) if there are signs of RICP.
— Keep temperature low normal (36–37 °C).
— Fluid restrict to 60% (0.9% saline) maintenance.

ACUTE PAIN MANAGEMENT: A QUICK GUIDE
Updated by Sabeena Qureshi, 2014
The analgesic ladder:

— A stepwise multimodal approach is important: Start with simple analgesic methods with few side effects progressing to sequential addition of other analgesics having greater effect but also additional side effects.

— Each drug should be given regularly at maximal doses.

— Local anaesthetic techniques should be used whenever possible.

— Assess the effectiveness of treatment and move up and down the analgesic ladder as necessary.

— Naloxone and anti-emetics must be prescribed if morphine is to be used, irrelevant of the route.

— Codeine has been omitted from the analgesic ladder for routine use.

The Analgesic Ladder

			*Tramadol PRN/ regular for age = ≥ 12y or dihydrocodeine	Oral morphine PRN or regular if needed	Systemic morphine (PCA/NCA) &/or epidural
	*NSAID regular	*NSAID regular	*NSAID regular	*NSAID regular	*NSAID regular
	Paracetamol regular	Paracetamol regular	Paracetamol regular	Paracetamol regular	Paracetamol regular
Nil	Mild	Mild to moderate	Moderate to severe	Moderate to severe	Severe

Mild pain: Paracetamol regular.

Mild to moderate: ADD NSAID* regular.

Moderate to severe: ADD Tramadol* PRN or regular if ≥12y or dihydrocodeine. If pain worsens, use oral morphine PRN or regularly. Antiemetics may be required with morphine.

Severe: Paracetamol and NSAID* regular with systemic morphine (PCA/NCA) and/or epidural.

Cautions:

*NSAIDs: <u>Contraindications</u>: Allergy, upper GI bleed, renal disease. Caution in thrombocytopaenia AND asthmatics. Patients may require gastric protection. Ask if NSAIDs are taken at home and tolerated. Diclofenac increases cardiovascular risks. Age restrictions: See further.

Paracetamol: Consider lower doses in liver failure (ask pharmacist).

Opiates: Reduce doses in renal impaiment/failure. They can cause respiratory depression and may cause nausea, vomiting and constipation.

*Tramadol: Only if >12y old. <u>Not advised</u> in cases with mucositis, transplantation or sickle cell crisis. Side effects: dysphoria, nausea, vomiting.

Children ≥1 month old:

Paracetamol:
— Oral 30 mg/Kg loading dose; 18 mg/Kg maintenance, 6 hrly regularly, maximum 75 mg/Kg/day, up to a max 4g/day.
— Rectal (poor absorption) 40 mg/Kg loading dose, 18 mg/Kg maintenance, 6 hrly regularly, maximum 75 mg/Kg/day, up to a max 4g/day.
— IV 6 hrly regularly; <10 Kg: 10 mg/Kg, max 30 mg/Kg/day; 10–50 Kg: 15 mg/Kg, max 60 mg/Kg/day; ≥50 Kg: 1g, max 4g/day.

Ibuprofen: Oral 7.5 mg/Kg, 6 hrly or 10 mg/Kg, 8 hrly, regularly, max 2.4 g/day and 600 mg/dose.

Diclofenac (age >6 m): Rectal/slow IV; 1 mg/Kg, 8 hrly regularly, max 150 mg/day.

Naproxen: Oral 5 mg/Kg, 12 hrly. Max 1 g/day.

Morphine sulphate oral: 4 hrly as required or regularly. 1–3 m: 50–100 microgr/Kg; 3–6 m: 100–150 microgr/Kg; 6 m–1y: 200 microgr/Kg; 1–2y: 200–300 microgr/Kg; >2 y: 200–400 microgr/Kg, max 20 mg per dose.

Morphine sulphate SC: 150 microgr/Kg, 4 hrly as required or regularly, max 20 mg per dose.

Morphine sulphate IV: 50–100 microgr/Kg, every 5–10 min as required but be careful to monitor respiratory rate, SaO_2, HR, BP and be ready to protect the airway and to ventilate if required.

Diamorphine (Intranasal): See diamorphine guidelines BNF(C).

Tramadol: Oral/slow IV. Age ≥12y: 50–100 mg, 4–6 hrly as required or regularly, max 400 mg/day. See comments above.

Antiemetics:

Ondansetron (first line): Oral/IV, 100 microgr/Kg, 8 hrly, max 4 mg per dose.

Cyclizine (second line): Oral/slow IV, 1 mg/Kg, 8 hrly, max 50 mg per dose.

Metoclopramide (third line): Oral/slow IV, 100 microgr/Kg, 8 hrly, max 10 mg per dose and max 0.5 mg/Kg/day, max 5 days.

Dexamethasone (fourth line): IV, 150 microgr/Kg, 8 hrly, max 8 mg per dose.

Naloxone:

FOR respiratory depression: **IV, 4 microgr/Kg, as required. Max 400 microgr.**

FOR pruritis/urinary retention: **IV, 0.5 microgr/Kg, as required. Max 50 microgr.**

Children <1 month old, >32 weeks gestation:

Paracetamol:
— Oral, 20 mg/Kg loading dose, 15 mg/Kg maintenance, 6 hrly, max 60 mg/Kg/day.
— PR, 30 mg/Kg loading, 20 mg/Kg maintenance, 8 hrly, max 60 mg/Kg/day.
— IV, 7.5 mg/Kg, 8 hrly, max 25 mg/Kg/day.

TRANSPORT OF THE CRITICALLY ILL CHILD: CATS GUIDELINES
Reviewed by Padmanabhan Ramnarayan, 2013

Refer to chapters relating to each diagnosis and to pages 9–21, 47, 183–187, 215.

Transport considerations when transfer undertaken by the local team:

— Discussion between the consultant of the retrieval service (CATS, for example) and the District General Hospital (DGH) consultant caring for the child to make an individual risk assessment. CATS consultant and the responsible DGH consultant should agree the transport plan jointly.

Initial stabilisation undertaken at the local DGH prior to transfer:

— Appropriate staff must be identified who are familiar with inter-hospital transfer and capable of managing the airway (includes usually an anaesthetist).
— Local ambulance service must be notified: State 'Time Critical Emergency Patient Transfer'.
— Airway must be secure.
— Copy of the chest X-ray must be available to take with team.

— Breathing: Ventilation adequate; end-tidal CO_2, blood gas.
— Circulation: Adequate fluid resuscitation given with sufficient IV access.
— Disability: BM, pupils, other focal neurological signs addressed.
— Family needs must have been addressed.
— Communication must take place with the receiving PICU via CATS. Notes must be photocopied.

Transport Considerations:

— Monitoring during transfer: ECG, SaO_2, BP (non-invasive or invasive), end-tidal-CO_2.
— Child sedated (morphine, midazolam infusions) and paralysed.
— ETT well secured/good position/no leak.
— Airway bag with tape, mask, T piece, ambubag, ETTs, laryngoscopes, all ready for an emergency.
— Drug bag prepared with fluid for boluses and resuscitation drugs ready for an emergency.
— Ventilator and sufficient oxygen.
— Adequate venous +/− arterial access.
— Infusion pumps for sedation, muscle relaxant, vasoactive infusions if required.
— Continuous infusions of sedation and muscle relaxant.
— Prepare and connect inotropes, ready to commence if required.

— Physiological targets: SaO_2 >95%, mean BP = target for age, end-tidal CO_2 4.5–5KPa.
— Choose other targets depending on the patient's condition.

CHILD ABUSE/PSYCHIATRY/DEATH

SUSPECTING CHILD ABUSE
www.nice.org.uk/nicemedia live/12183/44872/44872.pdf
Andrea Goddard and NICE Guidance on Child
Maltreatment, 2012

SUSPECT = serious concern about risk of child maltreatment:

Listen and observe: Any history that is given is important. Report of maltreatment, disclosure from a third party. Child's appearance, demeanour, behaviour. Symptoms and physical signs. Result of an investigation. Interactions between the parent/carer/child.

Seek explanations for any injury: Seek explanations from parent/carer and child/young person in a non-judgemental manner.

Unsuitable explanations: Implausible, inadequate, inconsistent with the child's presentation or activities, medical condition, age, developmental stage. Different accounts given by parent/carers and child. Different accounts over time. Accounts based on cultural practice.

Record everything: In the child's clinical record – what is observed and heard from whom and when. Record why this is of concern.

Contact: Senior A&E nurse, the paediatric site practitioner (PSP) and, during office hours, the consultant on call for child protection, or the general paediatric consultant. Out of hours, call the general paediatric consultant on call.

Alerting features – SUSPECT child maltreatment if:

Bruising: Observe the shape of a hand, ligature, stick, teeth, grip or implement.

Bruising or petechiae: If not caused by a medical condition, with an unsuitable explanation or in a child not independently mobile. Multiple or in clusters. Similar shape and size. On non-bony parts of face, body, eyes, ears, buttocks. On neck looking like attempted strangulation. On ankles and wrists looking like ligature marks.

Human bite marks are unlikely to have been caused by a young child and they are always suspicious.

Lacerations, abrasions: Scars that have unsuitable explanations or on a child not independently mobile. Multiple/ symmetrical. On areas protected by clothing. On eyes, ears, sides of face, neck, ankles and wrists that look like ligature marks.

Burn or scald injuries on a child: Unsuitable explanation. Not independently mobile. On soft tissue not expected to come into contact with a hot object (backs of hands, soles of feet, buttocks, back). In the shape of an implement (cigarette, iron etc.) that indicate forced immersion. Scalds to buttocks, perineum, lower limbs, limbs in a glove, stocking or symmetrical distribution or with sharply delineated borders.

One or more fractures in a child: **If there is no medical condition that predisposes to fragile bones (ex. osteogenesis imperfecta or osteopenia of prematurity) or if the explanation is absent or unsuitable. Fractures of different ages. X-ray evidence of occult fractures (ex. rib fractures in infants).**

Intracranial injury: **If there is no confirmed accidental trauma or known medical cause. Absent or unsuitable explanation? The child is aged under 3 years. There are also other inflicted injuries, retinal haemorrhages, rib or long bone fractures. Single/multiple subdural haemorrhages with or without subarachnoid haemorrhage with or without hypoxic ischaemic damage to the brain.**

Signs of spinal injury: **Injury to vertebrae or within the spinal canal. For example, cervical injury with inflicted head injury, or thoracolumbar injury with focal neurology or unexplained kyphosis. Spinal injury with no major confirmed accidental trauma.**

Intra-abdominal or intra-thoracic injury: **No major confirmed accidental trauma. Absent or unsuitable explanation. Delay in presentation. There may be no external bruising or other injury.**

Sexual abuse, neglect and/or emotional abuse: **Any concern about type of child abuse, contact the consultant on call for child protection and the general paediatric consultant.**

SAFEGUARDING CHILDREN AND YOUNG
PEOPLE TEAM

CHILD AND ADOLESCENT MENTAL HEALTH
SERVICE (CAMHS)
Contact details only:

<u>Mental Health problem identified:</u>

Non-self harm

Deliberate self harm

APPARENT LIFE THREATENING EVENTS (ALTE)

The Royal College of Pathologists and the Royal College of Paediatrics and Child Health, September 2004.
Prandota J. *American Journal of Therapeutics*, 2004, 11: 517–546.
Meadows R *Arch Dis Child*, 1999, 80: 7–14.

— Majority: <1 year old.
— 50% are 'idiopathic'.
— Those due to non-accidental injury (NAI) are of unknown frequency.

History: Ask the following questions:

— Pregnancy: This pregnancy and previous pregnancies? Maternal smoking?
  Birth history? IUGR?
— Parents: Related? Age, occupation, level of education, smoking, alcohol, drugs, medication?
— Child: On protection register? Neonatal life? Growth and development? Feeding, sleep (position, temperature, room), previous illness?
  Immunisations with date of last dose?
— History of event: Previous few days: Change in sleeping habit? Position (prone/supine)?
  Last 12–24 hours: Feeding? Temperature in room?
  When last seen? Position found in? Time of day? Any vomit? Colour change? What resuscitation manoeuvres? By whom?

Physical examination:

— Perform a complete examination including:
Dysmorphism, bruises, rash, petechiae, blood around mouth/nose, evidence of fractures, dehydration, pupils and fundi.

— Document any bruising or marks: **Draw a diagram of the child.**
— Fundi: **Inspect for retinal haemorrhages.**

Management: **Pages 9–21.**

— High flow O_2 (15L/min mask with reservoir bag) or intubation.
— Intubation (rapid sequence drugs): Page 183. Indicated if: GCS<8; unstable airway, respiratory distress, prolonged hypoxic-ischaemic insult with end organ damage.
— Monitor SaO_2, RR, BP, HR, end-tidal CO_2, blood gases.
  Perintubation: Beware of dropping BP. Is neuroprotection needed? Early fluid bolus? Inotropes? (Pages 47, 130, 216, 217.)
  If head trauma is suspected: <u>Oral</u> intubation + immobilise cervical spine + <u>oro</u>gastric tube if required (pages 130, 161).
— Circulation: Pulses, CRT, monitor HR, BP, base deficit, lactate, urine.
  Fluid bolus 10–20 ml/Kg 0.9% saline if hypovolaemia (pages 47, 216).

Central venous line or IO needle if peripheral access insufficient.

Maintain BP high normal if neuroprotection is needed (pages 130, 217, 218).

— Gastric tube on free drainage.

— Head midline and at 30°: If neuroprotection is needed (page 130).

— Blood tests: Arterial blood gas, electrolytes, urea, creatinine, troponine, bone profile, liver, BM, lactate, FBC and film, clotting, X-match.

— ET secretions, NPA (all respiratory viruses), per-nasal swab (pertussis), blood and urine cultures, chest X-ray.

— If signs of trauma: Immobilise cervical spine, full secondary survey, trauma X-rays, CT head/cervical spine if needed. Think of possible NAI. (Pages 161, 165, 201.)

— Organise a PICU transfer.

Special investigations:

As indicated by the history, physical examination and progress: <u>Blood:</u> glucose, anion gap, karyotype + store DNA, viral serology, toxicology. <u>Metabolic:</u> (blood carnitine, acyl-carnitine profile, amino acid profile, ammonia, lactate, pyruvate). <u>Urine:</u> Odour, ketones, organic and amino acids, reducing substances, toxicology. <u>Guthrie test</u> at birth if relevant. <u>Stool:</u> Microscopy, virology.

— As indicated, the following may be needed: Head US/CT/MRI, EEG, Skeletal survey, ECG, ECHO, Fundoscopy, pH study, Barium swallow, sleep study.

— CSF (if no contraindication to LP (page 124): Microscopy, gram stain, culture, PCR for infective pathogens, protein, glucose, lactate, pyruvate.
— Muscle and skin biopsy.
— Inform the child protection team and Social Services if there are concerns regarding non-accidental injury (NAI) (page 201).

DEATH OF CHILDREN: EXPECTED AND UNEXPECTED (UK Rules and Regulations)
Reviewed by Nelly Ninis, 2012

An unexpected death of a child is defined as follows: 'The death of a child that was not anticipated as a significant possibility 24 h before the death or where there was a similarly unexpected collapse leading to or precipitating the event that led to a death.'

It also covers children on PICU/NICU whose initial illness bringing them to critical care was unexpected. E.g. a child with meningitis who spends 5 days on PICU and develops brain stem death would be considered an *unexpected death* even though the death was inevitable and expected once the testing had been done because the reason for admission to PICU was unexpected.

In all *unexpected deaths and collapses*, non-accidental injury (NAI) and safety of the other children in the family must be considered. Do not wait for the child to die to consider this aspect of the case (page 201).

After all deaths:

— Complete the Trust Child Death pro forma.
— Form A needs to be sent to the SPOC (Single Point Of Contact for Child Death Overview Panel).
— Ensure form B (CDOP) is completed for every child death and for particular causes (SIDS, burns, drowning, traumatic injuries, etc...).

— Family liaison services should support all bereaved families both at time of death and weeks/months afterwards. The support should include that of siblings, facilitating viewings in the chapel for families and arrangements for some children/babies to go home after death if that is what families want and if there are no contraindications in doing so. It should also help organise follow up for all families at about 6 weeks post-death or later if a post mortem/inquest is needed.

— It is important that staff have a debrief session after dealing with a child or baby death to ensure that all staff can talk about the experience and support each other.

DRUGS

COMMONLY USED DRUGS IN THE FIRST
HOURS AND DOSES
Reviewed by Penny Fletcher, 2014

All drugs have side effects. Before giving any drug, you must know the risks, balance risks versus benefits and be prepared to troubleshoot if undesired effects occur.

<u>Approximate weight of children:</u> Weight in Kg:
— Previously advised formula: $(2 \times$ age years$)$ +4.
— More accurately: <12 m: $(0.5 \times$ age months$)$ +4; 1–5 y: $2 \times$ (age years) + 8; 6–12 y: $(3 \times$ age years$)$ +7.

Always refer to the current BNF(C) and to full guidelines.

<u>Nebulisers:</u>

Salbutamol: Preschool, <2 y: 2.5 mg; older: 5 mg.

Adrenaline 1/1000: Nebulised: 0.4 ml/Kg (max 5ml) in 3–5 ml 0.9% saline.

Atrovent (Ipratropium):
>5 y: 500 microgr; 1–5 y: 250 microgr; <1 y: 125 microgr.

3% saline: Use Muco Clear 3% saline nebules or prepare 1 ml NaCl 30% + 9 ml water for injection. Nebulise 4 ml + add salbutamol 1.25 mg (this lowers risks of airway hyper-reactivity) with 3% saline alone.

Budesonide: 2 mg nebulised.

Heliox: Page 37. A mixture of helium and oxygen that helps oxygen delivery to the alveoli; useful in upper airway obstruction and bronchiolitis. It can be used to drive nebulisers.

IV bronchodilators: **Page 38.**

Salbutamol: Requires SaO_2, BP, ECG monitoring.
IV bolus: <2y: 5 microgr/Kg, over 5–10 min, >2y: 15 microgr/Kg over 5–10 min (max 250 microgr).
Infusion: 10 mg salbutamol (=10 ml) added to 40 ml 0.9% saline/5% dextrose, 1–5 microgr/Kg/min = 0.3–1.5 ml/Kg/h.
Side effects: Lactic/metabolic acidosis, tachycardia, arrhythmias, tremor, hypokalaemia, hyperglycaemia, hypophosphataemia.

Magnesium sulphate: **40 mg/Kg over 20 min, max 2 g.** If using a 50% solution, dilute 5× in 0.9% saline. A 10% solution (10 g/100 ml) can be neat. Beware of dropping BP!

Aminophylline: Requires SaO_2, BP, ECG monitoring.
Loading dose: IV 5 mg/Kg (max 500 mg) over 20 min. Do not give if already receiving theophylline. Infusion: <9y: 1 mg/Kg/h; 9–16y: 0.8 mg/Kg/h. If <25Kg: Dilute 50 mg/Kg in 50 ml syringe dextrose or 0.9% saline; 1 ml/h = 1 mg/Kg/h. If >25 Kg: Dilute 500 mg in 500 ml.
Side effects: Arrhythmias, hypokalaemia, nausea, vomiting, dizziness.

Fluid boluses:

10–20 ml/Kg boluses (0.9% saline or 5% albumin). The indication is based on a complete clinical assessment: SaO_2, pulses, CRT, HR, BP, liver, heart (gallop, murmur) + blood gas (pH, lactate, base deficit).
Tricky: A rapid HR and long CRT can occur in situations where too much fluid can be dangerous: cardiac failure, DKA, RICP. So, <u>if the BP is acceptable,</u> it is important to take the time (60 sec) to <u>assess the CV system fully</u> before giving fluids, including assessment of the respiratory (pulmonary oedema?) and CNS (RICP?) systems (pages 9–21).

Saline concentrations:

0.9% saline = 0.9 g/100 ml = 150 mmol/L of NaCl.
1.8% saline = 1.8 g/100ml = 300 mmol/L of NaCl.
2.7% saline = 2.7 g/100ml = 460 mmol/L of NaCl.
3% saline = 3 g/100ml = 513 mmol/L of NaCl.
Ringer lactate 130 mmol/L.

Cardiovascular:

Adrenaline 1/10000 (=1 mg/10 ml) IV/IO for cardiac arrest: bolus; 0.1 ml/Kg = 0.01 mg/Kg = 10 microgr/Kg; IV, IO.
Anaphylaxis Adrenaline: See page 52
Adrenaline/Noradrenaline: IV centrally including IO; prepare 0.3 mg/Kg in 50 ml syringe 0.9% saline; 0.1 microgr/Kg/min= 1ml/h; start at 0.1 microgr/Kg/min, modify as need be. Infusions require continuous monitoring of SaO$_2$, BP, ECG.
Dopamine: IV peripherally or centrally including IO.
Prepare 3 mg/Kg in 50 ml syringe 0.9% saline; 5 microgr/Kg/min = 5 ml/h. Start at 5 microgr/Kg/min, increase as need be to 20 microgr/Kg/min.
Duct-dependent lesion: Page 83. Dinoprostone PGE2 (prostin).
Tetralogy of Fallot cyanotic spells: Page 86. Morphine, midazolam (buccal), esmolol, propanolol, metaraminol.

Arrhythmia:

Atropine for bradycardia: 10–20 microgr/Kg, IV.

SVT: Adenosine (page 79).

Amiodarone for SVT: IV; <1 m: 5 mg/Kg over 30 min; >1m: 5–10 mg/Kg (max 300 mg) over 20 min–2 h. Infusion: Call cardiologist (page 79).

Amiodarone for VF: 5 mg/Kg (max 300 mg) over at least 3min.

DC shock: <u>Cardioversion</u> in SVT 1–2 J/Kg, <u>defibrillation</u> 4 J/Kg (page 28).

<u>Pain/Sedation/Induction by anaesthetist:</u> **Pages 183–191.**

<u>Anticonvulsants:</u> **Page 123.**

Lorazepam **0.1 mg/Kg, max 4 mg; IV/IO. Risks of respiratory depression.**

Diazepam **rectally, nn:1.25–2.5 mg; 1 m–2 y: 5 mg; 2–12 y: 5–10 mg. Given IV increases risks of respiratory depression.**

Midazolam **buccal 0.3 mg/Kg. Risks of respiratory depression.**

Phenytoin **20 mg/Kg over 30 min; IV/IO.**

Phenobarbital **20 mg/Kg over 10 min, IV/IO.**

<u>Raised Intracranial Pressure (RICP):</u> **Page 130.**

Mannitol **20%=20 g/100 ml; IV 0.25 g/Kg over 15 min (can be repeated) to 1 g/Kg over 30 min. Beware of hypotension and low K^+ levels that will deteriorate cardiac function and reduce further the cerebral blood flow.**

3% saline for IV: **Take 36 ml out of a 500 ml bag 0.9% saline and replace with 36 ml of 30% saline. Alternatively use ready-made 2.7% saline bags. Give 3 ml/Kg over 5–10 min (page 217).**

Other:

Cetirizine PO: **Page 53.**

Cyclizine: **0.5–1 mg/Kg IV (pages 180, 193).**

Chlorphenamine: **Page 53.**

Dexamethasone: **0.15 mg/Kg, max 2 mg, IV, PO.**

Hydrocortisone: **1–4 mg/Kg, IV slow.**

Insulin infusion: **Page 150. Two different concentrations:**
— National guidelines and general paed wards:
  50 units in 50 ml 0.9% saline; 1 ml/h = 1 unit/h.
— For PICU: 5 units/Kg in 50 ml 0.9% saline; 1 ml/h = 0.1 unit/Kg/h.

Naloxone (Narcan®): **IV, IM, in ETT; 0.01 mg/Kg, repeated if** needed, max 2 mg. Then infusion of 0.01 mg/Kg/h (page 177).

Ondansetron: **0.1 mg/Kg by slow IV, PRN to 8 hrly. Max 4 mg/dose.**

Prednisolone: **1–2 mg/Kg, PO.**

Sugar for hypoglycaemia (<3 mmol/L): **10% dextrose; 2 ml/Kg, IV bolus; to be repeated if necessary (page 158).**

Sodium benzoate and phenylbutyrate: **Page 157.**

Tranexamic acid: **Page 173.**

Maintenance daily fluid requirements: **Page 95.**

Neonates: **150 ml/Kg/day.**

Infants 1–12 m: **100 ml/Kg/day.**

Older children:
— Up to 10 Kg: **100 ml/Kg/day.**
— 10–20 Kg: **Add to previous 50 ml/Kg/day for all additional Kg above 10 Kg.**
— 20–30 Kg: **Add to previous 20 ml/Kg/day for all additional Kg above 20 Kg.**
— >50 Kg: **2–2.5 litres per day.**

<u>Hypertension:</u> **Page 141.**

Nifedipine: 0.25–0.75 mg/Kg, oral/sublingual. Effect and length of action uncertain. Place IV access in case BP drops too fast.

Labetalol: 1–3 mg/Kg/h, continuous IV. Contraindications: asthma, cardiac failure.

Sodium nitroprusside: 0.5–8.0 microgr/Kg/min, continuous IV. Protect syringe from light.

Diazoxide: 2–10 mg/Kg, IV bolus.

Hydralazine: 0.1–0.2 mg/Kg, IV, IM.

Frusemide: 1–2 mg/Kg, IV. Only in presence of volume overload in acute renal failure or GN.

<u>Anti-poisons:</u> **Page 176.**

Naloxone (Narcan®): IV, IM, ETT. 0.01 mg/Kg, repeat to max 2 mg, then infusion 0.01mg/Kg/h.

<u>Antibiotics:</u> **Page 223 and refer to the BNF(C) and guidelines. Beware of renal dysfunction and dose modifications. Call a pharmacist.**

Aciclovir: For severe infections including neurological: IV, 3/d: IV <3m: 20 mg/Kg; 3m–12y: 500 mg/m^2; >12y: 10 mg/Kg.

Amoxicillin: IV, if <7d old: 100 mg/Kg, 2/d. If 7d–1m: same, 3/d; if >1m old: 50 mg/Kg, 6/d.

Azithromycin: PO 10 mg/Kg, per dose. 1/d for all ages.

Cefotaxime: IV, IM 50 mg/Kg per dose. 50 mg/Kg. If <7d old: 2/d. If 7–21d old: 3/d. If >21d old, 4/d.

Ceftriaxone: IV, IM 80 mg/Kg per dose, if >1m, 1/d.

Clindamycin: IV, if <14d old: 5 mg/Kg, 3/d. If 14d–1m: 5 mg/Kg, 4/d. If >1m: 10 mg/Kg, 4/d.

Gentamicin: IV, once a day. If >1m: 7 mg/Kg. If <1m: 5 mg/Kg. Max 450 mg/day. Renal dysfunction: Reduce to 2–5 mg/Kg depending on degree of dysfunction. Measure blood level 12 hours after dose.

Metronidazole: IV, 7.5mg/Kg, 3/d. (If <2m old: 2/d.)

Tazocin: IV 90 mg/Kg per dose, 4/d.

Vancomycin: IV, 8 hrly. If <1m: 15 mg/Kg per dose. If >1m: 20 mg/Kg per dose. Renal dysfunction: Reduce to 10 mg/Kg. Measure blood level 12–24 hours after dose.

Electrolyte corrections: $HCO3^-$, Na^+, K^+, Ca^{2+}, Mg^2:
Page 107.

SPECIFIC INFECTIOUS SYNDROMES

FIRST LINE TREATMENT
FOR SPECIFIC INFECTIOUS SYNDROMES
Hermione Lyall, Marianne Nolan, Penny Fletcher, 2014

— Always try to obtain appropriate clinical samples (blood, urine, CSF, joint fluid) before starting anti-infectives.
— Ceftriaxone*: If neonates have raised bilirubin levels or if they are severely unwell with shock and IV calcium may be given, cefotaxime should be used instead of ceftriaxone.
— Some cases <u>must</u> be referred to the Health Protection Agency (HPA).

<u>Neurological:</u>

Brain/epidural/spinal abscess:

— *S.aureus, Streptococcus sp.*, anaerobes, often polymicrobial, TB.
— Ceftriaxone* IV + metronidazole IV. Treat 6 weeks minimum.
— For spinal/epidural abscess or for MRSA cover, add IV vancomycin.
— Seek infectious disease specialist +/– neurosurgical advice.

Encephalitis /meningo-encephalitis: See page 126 for causes.

— Ceftriaxone* IV + aciclovir IV.
— If concurrent respiratory infection: Add azithromycin PO for Mycoplasma. Consider oseltamivir for Influenzae.
— If <3m: Add amoxicillin IV for *Listeria* species.

— Seek infectious disease specialist advice. Note travel history: TB? Malaria? Leptospirosis?

Meningitis: **Pages 65, 126.**

— If >3m: *N.meningiditis, S.pneumoniae, H.influenzae.* Consider TB. Ceftriaxone* IV + dexamethasone if suspected bacterial cause (CSF purulent, WCC >1000, high WCC + protein > 1g/L, or bacteria in gram stain). Give prophylaxis to close contacts if *N.meningiditis* or *H.influenza. N.meningiditis:* Treat 7 days; *H.influenzae:* Treat 10 days; *S.pneumonia:* Treat 14 days.
— If <3m: Group B Streptococcus, *E.coli, L.monocytogenes:* Ceftriaxone* IV (or cefotaxime) + amoxicillin IV: Treat at least 14 days.
— If Group B Streptococcus: Give prophylactic penicillin V until 6 months old.
— If neonatal Group B Streptococcus: Treat 14–21 days. If neonatal *E.coli:* Treat 21 days.
— If travelled outside the UK or if received prolonged courses of antibiotic therapy in the last 3 months: Add vancomycin (for resistant pneumococci).
— If gram positive bacilli on CSF: Add amoxicillin (for *Listeria*).
— If VP shunt or post neurosurgery: Coagulase negative *Staphylococcus, S.aureus, S.pneumonia* (CSF leak, basal skull fracture), gram negatives. Give ceftriaxone + vancomycin. Call neurosurgeons and infectious disease specialists.
— Contact prophylaxis (ciprofloxacin) for meningococcus or *H.influenzae.*
— Notify the HPA.

Eye:

Conjunctivitis:

Adenovirus, enterovirus, herpes simplex virus, *S.aureus, H.influenzae, M.catarrhalis.*
— Chloramphenicol eye ointment 1% qds.
— Consider also aciclovir eye ointment.
— Continue for 2 days after symptoms resolved.

Facial cellulitis including peri-orbital cellulitis:

Group A Streptococcus, *Streptococcus sp.*, *S.aureus, H.influenzae, M.catarrhalis,* anaerobes.
— Ceftriaxone* IV + metronidazole IV. Treat 10–14 days.
— Consider empirical MRSA cover: Add vancomycin.
— Seek ENT or ophthalmology advice.

Ophthalmia neonatorum:

— *N.gonorrhoea*: Usually during the first 5 days of life and bilateral with purulent discharge. Do URGENT gram stain. Ceftriaxone* IV. Treat 7 days.
— *C.trachomatis:* Usually at 5–14 days of life and with respiratory distress. Erythromycin PO. Treat 14 days.
— Ophthalmology emergency: Seek urgent opinion.
— Add topical eye care ½ hrly.
— Notify the HPA. Refer parents to a genito-urinary specialist.

ENT:

Otitis media:

Viral, *S.pneumoniae, H.influenzae, M.catarrhalis.*

— Co-amoxiclav duo PO or azithromycin if penicillin allergic. Treat 5 days.

Otitis externa with secondary infection:
P.aeruginosa, S.aureus, Aspergillus sp., Candida sp.

— Primary otitis: Gentisone HC®. Not if ear drum is perforated.
— Secondary otitis, after acute otits media or chronic suppurative otitis: Topical quinolones/aminoglycosides. Seek ENT opinion.

Epiglottitis /bacterial tracheitis: **Page 33.**
H.influenzae (HiB), *S.aureus, S.pneumoniae.*

— Ceftriaxone* IV. This is an EMERGENCY: Get urgent senior ENT + anaesthetic help.
— Notify the HPA. Give antibiotic prophylaxis for close contacts if HiB.

Cervical lymphadenitis:
Group A Streptococcus, *S.aureus, S.pneumoniae, H.influenzae (<5y), M.catarrhalis.*

— Co-amoxiclav PO/IV for 10 days or azithromycin if penicillin allergic for 3 days.

Sinusitis:
S.pneumoniae, H.influenzae, Streptococci, Staphylococci, anaerobes.

— Co-amoxiclav duo + metronidazole (if <10y) or doxycycline (if >10y). Treat 7–10 days. If pencillin allergy, give azithromycin for 3 days instead of co-amoxiclav.
— If there is eye involvement, treat as per the orbital cellulitis protocol.

Pharyngitis/tonsillitis/severe tonsillitis/quinsy:

Majority are viral including EBV. Also Group A Streptococcus, *Fusobacterium sp.*

— If <8y: Co-amoxiclav duo or azithromycin if penicillin allergic.
— If >8y: Penicillin V or azithromycin if penicillin allergic.
— If severe tonsillitis or quinsy or Lemierre's disease: IV Ceftriaxone* + metronidazole.
— Treat 10–14 days; 3 days for azithromycin.
— Consult ENT specialist if peri-tonsillar abscess, quinsy, retropharyngeal abscess.

Mastoiditis:

Group A Streptococcus, *S.aureus, S.pneumoniae,* anaerobes.
— Ceftriaxone* IV + metronidazole IV.
— Seek ENT advice + do a CT of mastoids: Mastoidectomy may be needed.

Lungs:

Bronchiolitis: **Page 35.**

RSV, adenovirus, influenza, parainfluenza, metapneumovirus.
— Antibiotics only if there is evidence of bacterial secondary infection.
— Consider BACH protocol (page 35).

Influenza A or B:

— If the child is unwell enough for hospital admission: Oseltamivir.
— Add co-amoxiclav PO/IV or ceftriaxone* IV. Treat 5 days.

Pneumonia:

S.pneumoniae, H.influenzae, Mycoplasma, *C.pneumoniae.*
Mixed viral + bacterial infection common. Consider TB.
— Mild: Co-amoxiclav duo if <5y.   Azithromycin
   if >5y or if penicillin allergy.
— Severe: Ceftriaxone* IV and treat 7 days + azithromy-
   cin PO and treat 3 days.

Empyema:

S.pneumoniae, Group A Streptococcus, *S.aureus, H.influenzae.*
— Ceftriaxone* IV + clindamycin IV. Treat a minimum of
   7 days.
— Chest drains may need to be placed: Seek advice from
   respiratory and radiology specialists.

Pertussis:

Bordetella pertussis, Bordetella parapertussis.
— Azithromycin PO 10 mg/Kg. Treat 5 days, all ages.
— Notify the HPA.

Heart:

Endocarditis:

S.aureus, S.epidermidis, alpha-haemolytic Streptococci,
Enterococci, *Coxiella sp.,* HACEK (*Haemophilus sp.,
Actinobacillus, Cardiobacterium, Eikenella, Kingella sp.*).
— Ceftriaxone* IV + vancomycin IV + gentamicin IV
   1 mg/Kg tds. Prolonged course.
— At least 3 blood cultures prior to antibiotics.
— Seek infectious disease and cardiology specialist advice.

Abdominal/gastro-intestinal:

Bloody diarrhoea:

E.coli (especially 0157), *Campylobacter, Salmonella* and *Shigella sp.*
— No treatment. Seek infectious disease specialist advice.
— Antibiotics may prolong bacterial excretion. Ciprofloxacin resistance is common.

Abdominal sepsis (including appendicitis or trauma): **Page 112.**
E.coli, gram negatives, Streptococci, Enterococci, anaerobes.
— Co-amoxiclav or ceftriaxone IV + gentamicin IV + metronidazole IV/PR. Treat 10 days.

Diarrhoea in hospital caused by *C.difficile*:
— Rare in children.
— Metronidazole PO. Treat 10 days.
— If possible stop other antibiotics.
— Seek infectious disease specialist advice.

Biliary sepsis/cholangitis:
E.coli, Enterobactereriaceae, Enterococci, occ anaerobes.
— Usually there is an underlying biliary atresia or liver failure.
— IV ceftriaxone* + IV vancomycin + consider metronidazole PO/IV/PR.
— Seek advice from a liver unit.

Renal/genito-urinary:

Urinary Tract Infection (UTI):

E.coli, Klebsiella sp., Proteus sp., Enterococcus sp.
— Cephalexin PO (except for *Enterococci*) or Co-amoxiclav duo PO.
— If penicillin allergy: Give nitrofurantoin initially.
— Treat 5–7 days. Culture results guide subsequent therapy.

Pyelonephritis / UTI with sepsis:

E.coli, Klebsiella sp., Proteus sp., Enterococcus sp., P.aeruginosa.
— Cefotaxime IV + gentamicin IV. Treat 14 days.
— *P.aeruginosa:* Piperacillin and tazobactam (Tazocin®) IV or ciprofloxacin if sensitive.
— Seek infectious disease specialist advice.

Pelvic Inflammatory Disease:

N.gonorrhoeae, Chlamydia sp., coliforms, anaerobes.
— If >12y, doxycycline PO+ metronidazole IV+ ceftriaxone* IV.
— Alternatives: Azithromycin, ofloxacin, cefixime.
— Seek gynaecology specialist advice.
— Consider child protection issues (pages 201–204).

Vaginal discharge in pre-pubertal girls:

C.albicans, Streptococcus sp.
— Co-amoxiclav duo + clotrimazole cream.
— Consider child protection issues (pages 201–204).

Sepsis and shock:

Sepsis: **Pages 47, 57, 59, 65.**

N.meningiditis, S.pneumoniae, S.aureus (+ PVL**),
H.influenzae, Klebsiella sp., Salmonella, other Gram negatives.
Listeria in neonates or immunocompromised. **PVL =
Panton–Valentine leukocidin toxin.

— If <3m: Ceftriaxone* IV + amoxicillin IV.
— If >3m: Ceftriaxone* IV +/- gentamicin IV.
— If vascular catheter *in situ*: Add vancomycin.
— If suspected toxic shock syndrome: Add IV clindamycin
  + IVIG.
— If suspected PVL *S.aureus:* Add IVIG + IV clindamycin +
  low molecular weight heparin.
— Seek infectious disease specialist advice.

Note travel history.

Febrile neutropenia: **Page 67.**

S.aureus, S.epidermidis, P.aeruginosa, Gram negatives, Fungi.
— Piperacillin and tazobactam (Tazocin®) + gentamicin IV.
— If penicillin allergy: Meropenem + gentamicin IV.
— Consider vancomycin if a Hickman line is *in situ.*
— Seek infectious disease and haematology specialist advice.

Bone/joint:

Septic arthritis: **Pages 73–76.**

S.aureus, Group A Streptococcus, *H.influenzae, S.pneumoniae,
Kingella kingae.*
— Ceftriaxone* IV + clindamycin IV/PO. Treat 2–3 weeks.
— Cultures prior to starting treatment if possible.
— Seek urgent orthopaedic opinion.

Osteomyelitis: **Pages 73–76.**

S.aureus (+PVL = Panton–Valentine leukocidin toxin), Group A Streptococcus, *H.influenzae, S.pneumoniae, N.meningitidis, Kingella kingae, Salmonella sp.* in sickle cell patients. Consider mycobacteria. Take specimens for cultures prior to starting treatment if possible.

— Ceftriaxone* IV + clindamycin IV/PO.
— Consider MRSA cover: Add vancomycin.
— Prolonged treatment (4–6 weeks).
— Seek urgent orthopaedic opinion.

Compound Fracture:

S. aureus, anaerobes, polymicrobial.

— Ceftriaxone* IV + metronidazole IV/PO.
— Prolonged treatment (4–6 weeks).

Skin/soft tissue:

Bites (human/animal):

Anaerobes, *S.aureus, Pasteurella sp.*

— Co-amoxiclav duo (discuss with specialist if penicillin allergic).
— Treat 7 days. Review tetanus status.

Necrotising fasciitis: **Page 63.**

Group A Streptococcus, *S.aureus, V.vulnificans, C.perfringens. B.fragilis.*

— Ceftriaxone* IV + clindamycin IV + consider gentamicin + IVIG.
— Add vancomycin if MRSA possible.
— Urgent surgical review required for all cases.

— Seek infectious disease specialist advice.
— Prolonged treatment.

Cellulitis/Impetigo/Infected eczema:

S.aureus, Group A Streptococcus +/– HSV (in eczema).

— If mild: Co-amoxiclav duo PO (clindamycin PO if penicillin allergic).
— If severe: IV clindamycin + gentamicin IV. Treat 10 days.
— Infected eczema: As above + aciclovir PO (IV if severe). Treat 5–7 days.
— Screen for MRSA.

<u>Penicillin allergy:</u>

Penicillins: Flucloxacillin, co-amoxiclav, piperacillin-tazobactam (Tazocin®).

Cephalosporins:

— Fewer than 1% of penicillin-allergic patients react to 3rd generation cephalosporins (ceftriaxone, cefotaxime, ceftazidime).
— For the 1st and 2nd generation cephalosporins, there is a significant risk of cross-reactivity (cefuroxime, cephalexin, cefaclor).

Carbapenems: Meropenem etc…

Though they share the beta-lactam structure of penicillins, the risk of cross-reactivity is very small even in penicillin-allergic patients.

NOTIFIABLE DISEASES

Health Protection (Notification) Regulations 2010:
http://www.hpa.org.uk/Topics/InfectiousDiseases/
InfectionsAZ/

— Acute encephalitis
— Acute infectious hepatitis
— Acute meningitis
— Acute poliomyelitis
— Anthrax
— Botulism
— Brucellosis
— Cholera
— Diphtheria
— Enteric fever (typhoid or paratyphoid fever)
— Epiglottitis–Bacterial tracheitis
— Food poisoning
— Haemolytic uraemic syndrome (HUS)
— Infectious bloody diarrhoea
— Invasive Group A Streptococcal disease
— Legionnaires' disease
— Leprosy
— Malaria
— Measles
— Meningitis (bacterial)
— Meningococcal septicaemia
— Mumps
— Ophthalmia neonatorum
— Pertussis

First Line Treatment for Specific Infectious Syndromes

— Plague
— Rabies
— Rubella
— SARS
— Scarlet fever
— Smallpox
— Tetanus
— Tuberculosis
— Typhus
— Viral haemorrhagic fever (VHF)
— Whooping cough
— Yellow fever

GENERAL INFORMATION

GROWTH CHARTS — BOYS (WHO/RCPCH): 0–4 YEARS OLD

World Health Organisation 2006: Child Growth Standards for healthy, breastfed children: www.rcpch.ac.uk/growthcharts

Measurements must be written on growth charts.

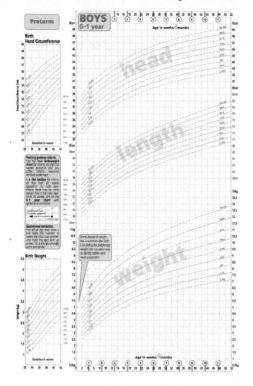

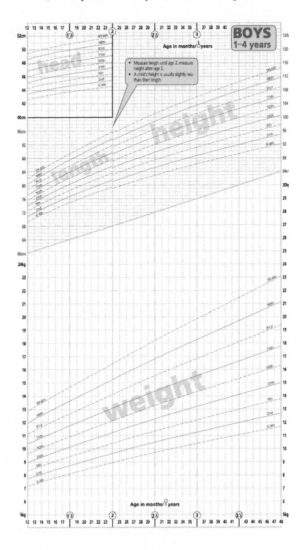

GROWTH CHARTS — GIRLS (WHO/RCPCH): 0–4 YEARS OLD

World Health Organisation (WHO) 2006: Child Growth Standards for healthy, breastfed children: www.rcpch.ac.uk/growthcharts

Measurements must be written on growth charts.

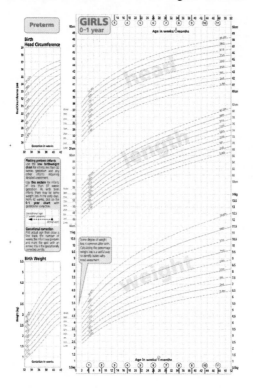

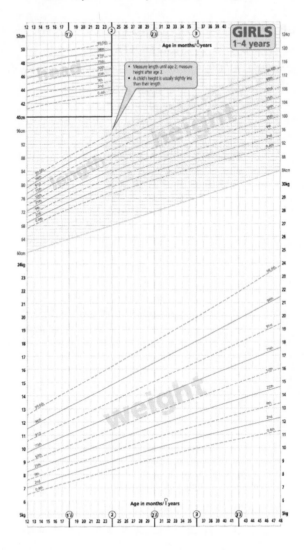

BODY MASS INDEX (BMI)
Scientific Advisory Committee on Nutrition and the Royal College of Paediatrics and Child Health in April 2012.
National Centre for Health Statistics and the National Centre for Chronic Disease Prevention and Health Promotion, 2000: http://www.cdc.gov/growthcharts

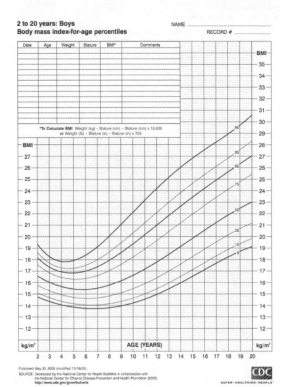

BMI calculation: weight (Kg) / [height (m)]^2

BMI calculators:

— http://www.nhs.uk/tools/pages/healthyweightcalcula-tor.aspx?WT.mc_id=101007
— http://www.nhs.uk/Tools/Pages Healthyweightcalculator.aspx

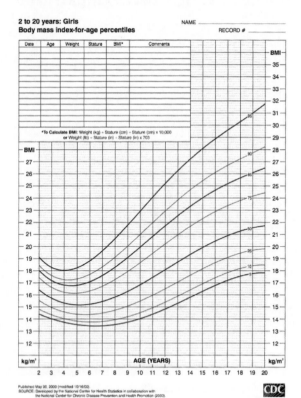

2 to 20 years: Girls
Body mass index-for-age percentiles

ESTIMATING BODY SURFACE AREA

Age	Estimated Weight (Kg)	Estimated Surface Area (m^2)
Newborn	3.5	0.25
3m	6	0.3
6m	7	0.38
9m	9	0.45
1y	10	0.5
3y	14	0.6
5y	17	0.75
7y	20	0.9
10y	30	1
12y	40	1.3
14y	50	1.5
16y+	60 – 65 – 70	1.60 – 1.75 – 1.8

SOME USEFUL FORMULAS

Anion gap:
$(Na^+ + K^+) - (Cl^- + HCO3^-)$

BMI calculation:
Weight (Kg)/height (m^2)

Corrected Na$^+$ in hyperglycaemia:
Measured Na$^+$ + [1.6 × (blood glucose − 5.5)/5.5]

Osmolar gap:
$2Na^+$ + urea + glucose − measured osmolarity

Replacement for dehydration:
% dehydration × weight (Kg) × 10 = fluid deficit in ml. Add to maintenance volume.

Serum osmolality:
Normal = 270–295 mosm/L
$[2 × (Na^+ + K^+)]$ + blood glucose + urea.

Water deficit (ml) in hypernatraemia:
Water deficit = 4 ml/Kg for each 1mmol/L serum Na$^+$ over 145 mmol/L.

Weight of children age 1–12 years (Kg):
Previously advised formula: 2 × (age years + 4).
Current recommended formula:
<12m: 0.5 × (age months) + 4;
1–5y: 2 × (age years) + 8;
6–12y: 3 × (age years) +7.

UNIT CONVERSIONS AND DOSE CALCULATION

Paediatric dose calculator:
http://www.medcalc.com/pedidose.html

Volumes:
1 gallon = 4546 ml
1 pint = 568.26 ml
1 fluid ounce = 28.41 ml
1 cubic centimetre = 1 g = 1 ml (approximately)
1 tablespoon = 15 ml (approximately)
1 teaspoon = 5 ml (approximately)
15–16 drops = 1 ml (approximately)

Weights:
1 lb (pound) = 0.45 Kg
1 Kg = 2.2 lb
1 stone = 6.35 Kg
1000 microgram = 1 mg

Temperature:
°F = (°C × 1.8) + 32

Length:
1 foot = metre ÷ 3.2808
1 inch = centimetre × 0.3937

Concentrations:
1:100 = 1 g/100 ml = 1%
1:1000 = 1 g/1000 ml = 1 mg/ml = 0.1%
1:10000 = 1 g/10000 = 1 mg/10 ml = 0.01%

International units (IU):

Old measurement of vitamin activity determined by biological methods.

New measures are determined by chemical analysis.

Health foods and supplements still use IU.

Vitamin A: 1 IU = 0.3 microgr retinol, 3.6 microgr b-carotene, or 7.2 microgr other vitamin A carotenoids.

Vitamin D: 1 IU = 0.025 microgr colecalciferol.

Vitamin E: 1 IU = 0.67 microgr natural a-tocopherol.

REFERENCES AND FURTHER READING

General Information:

— APLS 2012.
— ATLS 2010.
— Resuscitation Council (RC) 2010.
— European Resuscitation Council (ERC) 2010.
— *Rogers Textbook of Paediatric Intensive Care*, 4th ed., Williams and Wilkins, 2008.
— South Thames Retrieval Service (STRS).
— Children Acute Transport Service (CATS).
— Great Ormond Street Hospital (GOSH).
— National Institute for Health and Clinical Excellence (NICE).

Airway Management:

— Intubation and airway management. STRS Guidelines, 2007.
— Intubation. CATS Guidelines, 2011.
— Pre-transport stabilisation. STRS Guidelines, 2007.
— Anaesthesia in infants and children. GOSH Guidelines, 2006.
— Securing oral ETT. STRS Guidelines, 2007.

Anaphylaxis:

— Muraro. The management of anaphylaxis in child-hood: Position paper of the European academy of allergology and clinical immunology. *Allergy*, 2007, 62 (8): 857–887.

— Emergency treatment of anaphylactic reactions. Resuscitation Council, 2010.

— NICE Anaphylaxis Guidelines, 2011.

Asthma:

— British Guidelines on the Management of Asthma, British Thoracic Society, 2012.

— RCPCH: Allergy Care Pathway for Children, 2011.

— GINA: Pocketbook Guide for Allergy Management and Prevention, 2014.

— Breathing Difficulty: An evidence-based guideline for the management of children presenting with acute breathing difficulty. Paediatric Accident and Emergency Research Group, 2002.

Bronchiolitis:

— Bronchiolitis in children. Scottish Intercollegiate Guidelines Network, 2006.

— Bronchiolitis. CATS Guidelines, 2011.

— Breathing Difficulty: An evidence-based guideline for the management of children presenting with acute breathing difficulty. Paediatric Accident and Emergency Research Group, 2002.

Burns:

— Hettiaratchy. Initial management of a major burn: II — assessment and resuscitation. *BMJ*, 2004, 10, 329(7457): 101–103.

— Walker. Fluid Resuscitation of Childhood Burns: Paediatric. CoBIS Guidelines, 2009.
— Burns. CATS Guidelines, 2009.
— London and South East England Burn Network (LSEBN), 2010.

Cardiac: SVT, Duct-Dependent Diseases, Fallot Tetralogy:

— ERC guidelines, 2010.
— American Heart Association Guidelines, 2010.
— International Consensus on Cardiopulmonary Resuscitation and Emergency Cardiovascular Care Science with Treatment Recommendations (COSTR), 2010.
— London Kent Surrey & Sussex Duct-Dependent Congenital Heart Disease: Review, 2008.
— Shekerdemian. Management of the neonate with symptomatic congenital heart disease. *Arch Dis Child Fetal Neonatal*, 2001, 84: F141–F145.
— Starship Paediatric Cardiology Guidelines, Auckland, 2010. www.adhb.govt.nz / starshipclinicalguidelines.
— *The Pediatric Cardiology Handbook*, Mosby, 2003.
— *Pediatric Cardiac Intensive Care*, Williams and Wilkins, 1998.
— *Pediatric Acute Care*, 2nd ed., Williams and Wilkins, 2001.

Croup/Upper Airway Obstruction:

— Guideline for the diagnosis and management of croup. Toward Optimized Practice (TOP), Alberta Medical Association, 2007.

— Croup. The Royal Hospital for Sick Children, Yorkhill Guidelines, 2011.
— Acute Upper Airway Obstruction: Clinical Practice Guidelines. The Royal Children's Hospital, Melbourne, 2012.
— Upper Airway Obstruction. CATS Guideline, 2011.

Diabetic Ketoacidosis:

— Savage. Diabetes UK Position Statements and Care Recommendations, Joint British Diabetes Societies guidelines for the management of diabetic ketoacidosis, 2011.
— DKA. STRS Guidelines, 2008.
— DKA. CATS Guidelines, 2011.
— Rosenbloom. The management of diabetic ketoacidosis in children. *Diabetes Ther*, 2010, 1(2): 103–120.

Endocrine:

— Donaldson. Presentation, acute illness, and learning difficulties in salt wasting 21-hydroxylase deficiency. *Arch Dis Child Fetal and Neonatal Ed*, 1994, 70(3): 214–218.

Gastroenteritis:

— Gastroenteritis in children — Treatment. NHS Choices, 2012. www.nhs.uk/Conditions/Rotavirus-gastroenteritis/Pages/Treatment.aspx
— Szajewska. Management of acute gastroenteritis in Europe and the impact of the new recommendations:

a multicenter study. The Working Group on acute Diarrhoea of the European Society for Paediatric Gastroenterology, Hepatology, and Nutrition. *J Pediatr Gastroenterol Nutr*, 2000, 30(5): 522–527.

— Guandalini. Treatment of acute diarrhea in the new millennium. *J Pediatr Gastroenterol Nutr*. 2000, 30: 486–489.

Growth Charts and BMI Chart:

— World Health Organisation: Child Growth Standards for healthy, breastfed children, 2006. www.rcpch.ac.uk/growthcharts

— Scientific Advisory Committee on Nutrition and the Royal College of Paediatrics and Child Health, April 2012.

— National Centre for Health Statistics and the National Centre for Chronic Disease Prevention and Health Promotion, 2000. http://www.cdc.gov/growthcharts

Head Injury:

— Head injury: Triage, assessment, investigation and early management of head injury in infants, children and adults. NICE, 2007.

— Time Critical Neurosurgical Transfer. STRS Guidelines, 2010.

— Neurosurgical Emergency. CATS Guidelines, 2011.

— Head Injury Guideline; Clinical Practice Guidelines. The Royal Children's Hospital, Melbourne, 2013.

— Guidelines for the Acute Medical Management of Severe Traumatic Brain Injury in Infants, Children, and Adolescents, 2nd Ed., *Pediatr Crit Care Med*, 2012, 13, 1(Suppl): S1–82.

Infectious & Inflammatory Diseases: Kawasaki, Toxic Shock Syndrome:

— *Principles & Practice of Pediatric Infectious Diseases*, 4th ed., Elsevier, 2012.
— Sakata *et al.* A randomised prospective study on the use of 2 g IVIG or 1 g IVIG as therapy for Kawasaki disease. *Eur J Pediatr*, 2007, 166(6): 565–571.
— Ferguson. Gram-positive toxic shock syndromes. *Lancet Infect Dis*, 2009, 9(5): 281–290.
— Eleftheriou *et al.* Management of Kawasaki Disease. *P Arch Dis Child*, 2014, 99(1): 74–83.
— Kobayashi *et al.* Efficacy of immunoglobulin plus prednisolone for prevention of coronary artery abnormalities in severe Kawasaki disease (RAISE study): a randomised, open-label, blind-endpoints trial. *Lancet*, 2012, 28:379(9826): 1613–1620.

Malaria:

— Reyburn. New WHO guidelines for the treatment of malaria. *BMJ*, 2010, 340: c2637.
— Lubell *et al.* Cost-effectiveness of parenteral artesunate for treating children with severe malaria in sub-Saharan Africa. *Bull World Health Organ*, 2011, 89: 504–512.
— Maitland. Mortality after fluid bolus in African children with severe infection. *NEJM*, 2011, 26: 2483–2495.

Meningitis/Encephalitis:

— Sáez-Llorens. Bacterial meningitis in children. *Lancet*, 2003, 361(9375): 2139–2148.
— Tunkel. Practice Guidelines for the Management of Bacterial Meningitis. *Clinical Infectious Diseases*, 2004, 39(9): 1267–1284.
— Management of Bacterial Meningitis in Children and Young People, 2010. www.meningitis.org/assets/x/53067
— Feverish illness guideline CG47. NICE, 2007. www.nice.org.uk/cg047

Meningococcal Disease:

— Meningococcal Disease Algorithm, Meningitis Research Foundation: Meningitis & Septicaemia. www.meningitis.org
— Pollard. Emergency management of meningococcal disease: eight years on. *Arch Dis Child*, 2007, 92: 283–286.
— Thompson, Levin. Clinical recognition of meningococcal disease in children and adolescents. *Lancet*, 2006, 367 (9508): 397–403.
— Welch *et al.* Treatment of meningococcal infection. Community child health, public health, and epidemiology. *Arch Dis Child*, 2003, 88: 608–614.
— Visintin *et al.* Management of bacterial meningitis and meningococcal septicaemia in children and young people: summary of NICE guidance. *BMJ*, 2010, 28 (340): c3209.

— Dellinger. Surviving Sepsis Campaign: International Guidelines for Management of Severe Sepsis and Septic Shock. *Int Care Med*, 2008, 34(1): 17–60.
— Pathan *et al.* Pathophysiology of meningococcal meningitis and septicaemia. *Arch Dis Child*, 2003, 88(7): 601–607.

Metabolic Diseases:

— Metabolic Disorders. The Royal Children's Hospital, Melbourne, 2012.
— British Inherited Metabolic Disease Group, 2008. www.bimdg.org.uk
— Auron, Brophy. Hyperammonaemia in review: pathophysiology, diagnosis and treatment. *Pediatr Nephrol*, 2012, 27: 207–222.

Myocarditis:

— Triposkiadis. Diagnosis and Management of Myocarditis. International Seminar: New Insights in Cardiomyopathies. Thessaloniki, June, 2011.

Necrotising Fasciitis:

— Ustin. Necrotising soft tissue infections. *Crit Care Med*, 2011, 39(9): 2156–2162.
— Sultan. Necrotising fasciitis. *BMJ*, 2012, 345: e4274.
— Hashan. Necrotising fasciitis. *BMJ*, 2005, 330: 830–833.

Nephrology:

— Andreoli. Acute kidney injury in children. *Pediatr Nephrol*, 2009, 24: 253–263.
— The child with acute renal failure. Clinical Paediatric Nephrology, 3rd ed., Oxford University Press, 2003.
— Lurbe. Management of high blood pressure in children and adolescents: recommendations of the European Society of Hypertension. *J Hypertens*, 2009, 27: 1719–1742.

Neurology: Epilepsy, RICP:

— Pediatric Status Epilepticus: treatment and management. emedicine medsacpe.com, 2011.
— *Rogers Textbook of Paediatric Intensive Care*, 4th ed., Williams and Wilkins, 2008.
— Dunn. Raised intracranial pressure. *J Neurol Neurosurg Psychiatry*, 2002, 73(Suppl 1): i23–i27.
— Status epilepticus. STRS Guidelines, 2008.
— Febrile Convulsion: Clinical Practice Guidelines. The Royal Children's Hospital, Melbourne, 2012.

Osteomyelitis/Septic Arthritis:

— Cunnington. Severe invasive Panton–Valentine Leukocidin positive Staphylococcus aureus infections in children in London. *J Infect*, 2009, 59: 28–36.
— Pääkkönen. Management of a child with suspected acute septic arthritis. *Arch Dis Child*, 2012, 97(3): 287–992.

— Peltola. Short- versus long-term antimicrobial treatment for acute hematogenous osteomyelitis of childhood: prospective, randomized trial on 131 culture positive cases. *Pediatr Infect Dis J*, 2010, 29(12): 1123–1128.

— Faust *et al.* Managing bone and joint infection in children. *Arch Dis Child*, 2012, 97(6): 545–553.

Pain Management:

— Treatment of Acute Pain in children in the Emergency Department. Guidelines for the management of pain in children. The College of Emergency Medicine, Best Practice Guidelines, 2013.

Pharmacy:

— BNF(C) June 2014.
— Nelson's Pediatric Antimicrobial Therapy 19th Edition.
— Imperial Trust Neonatal Vade Mecum 2014.

Safeguarding and ALTE:

— When to suspect child maltreatment. National Collaborating Centre for Women's and Children's Health. NICE, 2009. www.nice.org.uk/nicemedia live/12183/44872/44872 and 44954. pdf.

— Prandota. Possible Pathomechanisms of Sudden Infant Death Syndrome. *Am J Ther*, 2004, 11: 517–546.

— Meadows. Unnatural Sudden Infant Death. *Arch Dis Child*, 1999, 80: 7–14.

INDEX

SOME BLEEPS AND TELEPHONE NUMBERS

Hospital Switchboard
Emergency

Allergy

Anaesthesia

Burn Services

Cardiologists

Dermatology

Diabetes

Endocrinology

ENT

Family Liaison Sister

Gastroenterology

General Paediatrics

Genetics

Gynaecology

Haematology

HIV

Immunology

Maxillofacial surgery

Mental Health Service

Metabolic specialist

Nephrology

Neurology

Neurosurgery

Ophtalmology

Orthopaedics

Paediatric surgery

Paediatric Site Practitioner (PSP)

Paediatric Transport Service

Pharmacy

PICU

Plastic surgery

Respiratory disease specialists

Safeguarding

Tissue viability

TOXBASE **National Poisons Information Service**
24h poisons information in the UK: 0844 8920111
Office: +44 (0) 131 2421383

Urology

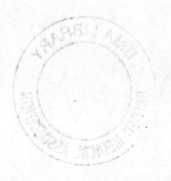

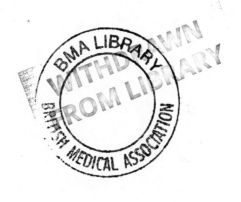